ROCK STAR

My Triumph over Guillain Barre' Syndrome

Fr. Dave Barrett

MCP

Fr. Dave Barrett has been a priest for twenty years. This is his first book, but he really enjoys writing and public speaking. He writes a weekly column for his church bulletin for his parish the New Prague Area Catholic Community in New Prague, Minnesota. He serves as the Regional Associate Pastor. He writes a weekly blog entitled Second Hand Preacher attached to the parish website (npcatholic.org). There is also a monthly newsletter he has a column in for the Knights of Columbus in New Prague. He enjoys celebrating mass at St. John's the Evangelist Church in Union Hill, and St. Scholastica in Heidelberg. He also has regular masses in several other communities.

The author earned a BS in Food Science from the University of Wisconsin-River Falls. He worked for four years in the food industry before entering the seminary. He was awarded a Master of Divinity from the St. Paul Seminary at the University of St. Thomas in St. Paul, Minnesota. Fr. Dave served as a priest in the St. Paul metro for eight years before coming to the Montgomery/New Prague area twelve years ago.

Fr. Dave grew up in Randolph Minnesota on a diversified crop and livestock farm with his parents, along with his much younger two brothers and two sisters. His parents are still on the farm and he gets there quite a bit. Father enjoys, good books, movies and an occasional Netflix binge. He loves animals, especially his cat Miriam.

Mill City Press, Inc.
2301 Lucien Way #415
Maitland, FL 32751
407.339.4217
www.millcitypress.net

© 2017 by Fr. Dave Barrett

Printed in the United States of America

ISBN-13: 978-1-54561-658-1

For my family—blood and church—especially my sister Joan: without all you I couldn't have made the journey.

Table of Contents

Foreword

It seems like a nightmare, something we imagine happens to someone else, not someone we know and care about. It was a busy active day, enjoying time with family when the next day my brother found himself calling 911 and two days after that, nodding his approval to be placed on a ventilator. Diagnosed with a rare neurological disease, Guillain Barre Syndrome, my brother lay in a hospital bed unsure of what would happen, but knowing his life would forever be changed.

As a medical social worker, I have worked with many patients and families as they face difficult medical situations. I certainly recognized their struggle, but never truly knew what they might be feeling or thinking... the fear, the worry, the wonder of where God is in the midst of this struggle. I walked the journey alongside my brother, gained my own insights, but until reading this book- Rock Star- I never really understood all that he went through. Through story and reflection, one rides a rollercoaster of emotion as he chronicles his months of recovery. From the story of being chased by a monster that shook his heavily sedated dreams to the fear of not being able to communicate due to a weak voice and limbs to the heartwarming triumph of taking his first steps and being called "rock star" by his physical therapist, the stories offer insight into something most of hopefully will never experience.

Yet there is something more. My brother, as a Catholic priest, is often the one giving support and encouragement to those dealing with difficult times. During his illness, he had to accept care, prayers, and support from so many others. He writes "disease breaks us apart. We feel alone in illness and we need reconnection… One of the gifts of GBS is that I have learned how I can depend on others. I don't have to do everything myself." Using well-chosen scripture passages and reflections on his own journey with God, readers gain insight in ways to grow closer to God in the midst of struggle and ways to humbly accept the love of those around us. And though we all certainly hope and plan to avoid a major medical event, life comes with challenges that we must face. The important thing is that we can work on gaining the tools to face those challenges.

Joan Hlas

September 25, 2017

Acknowledgments

I would like to thank all those who gave me medical care during my three month hospitalization. This includes the doctors and staff at Methodist Hospital in St. Louis Park, Minnesota. This is where I received the most critical care. I was transferred to Regency Hospital where I received step down treatment and had some amazing recovery. I also want to thank the doctors, therapists and staff at Courage Center (now Courage Kenney Institute) in Golden Valley where I received great rehabilitation

Writing the book was a long and exhaustive process. I couldn't have done it without Mary Carol Moore of the Loft Literary Center in Minneapolis. I took four on-line classes with her as my instructor. I also want to thank the many students whom I shared parts of my writing which includes Lucy Rose and Susan Chandler who were among the most helpful. I am thankful for friends who did some reading along the way. I'm also thankful to the many coffee shops I wrote in.

I want to especially thank one of my parishioners, Olivia Lemke who designed the cover of my books. She is a student in graphic design and did an outstanding job.

The people at Mill City Press who are a division of Salem Publishing worked with me to bring this book alive. I would like to thank Krystle Prashad, Elizabeth Marrero and Jose Medina along with the rest of the staff.

I would like to thank my sister Joan Hlas for her direction of my medical care and for writing the forward of this book. My family was very supportive with this project and I am filled with gratitude.

Most of all I would like to thank the Triune God that gives me strength. The Father who gives me the creative spark to do all the projects in my life. I thank Jesus for his companionship along the way as I deal with life's obstacles. I want to thank the Holy Spirit for the motivation to put this project together. The Holy Spirit is my guide as I serve God and the people in my care as I humbly live my life as a Catholic Priest.

Chapter 1

Blue Angel

Then Peter recovered his senses and said, "Now I know for certain that the Lord has sent an angel and rescued me" (Acts 12:11).

I opened my eyes and saw light, wondering if this was another dream. There was an incredible warmth in my body that felt almost suffocating, and the whole room was a little uncomfortable. I scanned the room and saw mostly bare walls along with a sterile white ceiling over me. There were parts of several IVs above my head, and I noticed a line going to a port just above my left hand. I tried to lift my hand, but it wouldn't move. Panic started to set in. I tried my other — nothing. Soon I realized there was no movement in my legs, either, and I thought *I am in real trouble*. Trapped in that bed, I tried to thrash around with my head and a bit of my torso, but there was little movement.

Just then I heard some ear-popping beeping going on above my head. The noise was so loud, that anxiety built up within me. Suddenly there was a whoosh of air, and I heard a door opening.

"Dave, it's okay," said an attractive woman with her beautiful face. She looks like an angel. Have I died and gone to heaven? I'm not certain what heaven is like; could this be it? Looking at her comforted me, and I temporarily forgot that I couldn't move. She was no chubby cherub from the Old Italian paintings I had seen that my racing mind tried to compare her to. Instead she was dressed all in blue, a dark blue, which gave her a majestic look. Maybe this was a dream and she was some sort of blue angel without wings. The melodic sound of her voice calmed me down, and for the moment I believed her that somehow my situation was okay.

"Dave, you might not remember, but you are in Methodist hospital, and you have been very sick. For your own safety, you need to stay calm and try and lay peacefully."

I wanted to be anywhere but here, so my focus was on her angelic face. Her voice seemed to match some of the expectations of what I believed an angel would sound like. The sound was pleasant, and my heart was hopeful. For a moment everything seemed so surreal. I wanted her to be an angel because if she was, that might mean that none of this was real. I wanted to wake up to my alarm where I could have risen from bed slowly to greet another day. Instead I was in this preconscious state, being told I was in a hospital room.

So this probably wasn't a dream or some sort of heavenly realm. Suddenly I remembered having Guillian Barre Syndrome (GBS) pronounced Gee Yon Ber Ray, in which the brain receives inappropriate signals that result in tingling, "crawling-skin," or painful sensations. Because the signals to and from the arms and

2

legs must travel the longest distances, they are most vulnerable to interruption. Therefore, muscle weakness and tingling sensations usually first appear in the hands and feet. GBS is a disease of the central nervous system affecting communication between the brain, the spinal cord, and the nerves that extend to the trunk and limbs.

Being really scared, I prayed a short prayer of hope, asking Jesus to be with me in this tough spot. I knew in my mind that most people live, but I was scared that I wouldn't get back to normal. I couldn't move, and that couldn't be good. I wanted to know if I was normal, so then I try to respond.

"I can't move. Is this normal?" That was what I thought I was said, but the sound came out, "Blah, blah, blah." I sounded like one of the adults in an old *Peanuts* cartoon special.

"I can't understand you as you have a trach to help you breathe," said the nurse.

I wondered what that was, but she pointed to her neck, and I noticed a tube in my neck. The blue angel is right; I am not talking so that anyone can understand.

"I'm Amy, and I will be your nurse. I'm not going anywhere. I'll check on you constantly. All you need to do is stay calm and sleep if you can. You'll heal faster if you sleep, and we are giving you medication to help you do so."

As a reflex, I try a quick "Thank you," but all that came out was another "blah."

I trusted her, and she calmed me down, but I was scared and wondered how this was going to play out. Would I talk again? Move again? I heard that others who had Guillian Barre Syndrome survived. I would get better, wouldn't I? But for now I had almost no movement and no way to communicate.

Where is God in this? I had been a Catholic priest for fifteen years; shouldn't I know? As a priest, I was so independent. I expressed to others their need for God. I had helped countless people with problems like divorce, abuse, death, and so many other circumstances. I was now the needy one. Being full of doubt, I tried to think positive thoughts. I realized in that moment of pity that I was still alive and had a better than decent chance of living.

Besides, God was sending me an angel in the form of this nurse. Angels are messengers, and Amy was telling me to lie peacefully rather than ask all of these tough questions. Perhaps this angel could help me in my life journey. I was scared because I couldn't comprehend being this sick. For now fear was still my constant companion. I felt warm air on my cheeks, and there was that aseptic hospital smell in the air that made me feel sick and uncomfortable. I was forced to lie here with my emotions. I felt stuck both physically and emotionally.

Could I trust Amy the angel, or was she just sent to keep me calm? I was exhausted, but I couldn't sleep. I had to live with these unanswered questions, and this would take some getting used to. I liked things sort of predictable, but I was going into a great unknown. I was trapped in my body!

Chapter 2

The Wild Ride

"My God my God why have you abandoned me, why so far off from my cry for help." (Psalm 22:2)

A few days before I met the Blue Angel was when the story really began. I felt weird on Wednesday and went to bed with tingling hands and feet. The feeling was like alien weird, similar to the sensation you get when foot falls asleep, but it didn't go away. On Thursday I awoke to much the same. I just felt tired, and there was this pulsating sensation in my body. I wondered if I should I stay home. That twelve-day trip I had just gotten back from seemed like motivation to get back to work. I hated to be gone that long. Was I poised to go out into the world? If only I could have buttoned this shirt. Because of the struggle, I went for every other button. Running late, I gulped a sip of milk and took my pills. Everything seemed to be in slow motion. I had morning mass, and with the way I felt, it was sure to be an adventure.

The Church at St. Wenceslaus was large and ornate with beautiful stained-glass windows. Because it is so large, people were spread out all over. I was so far away from them that they looked like colorful dots on a sea of brown pews. I wore a beautiful green vestment and felt the warmth of the lights shining down on me.

I was nervous because my physical condition was failing me. I prayed that I could stay upright at mass. I guess I preached. I only remembered just trying to get through the mass. I had celebrated mass several thousand times. Each one was special, even this one I struggled at. Jesus gave us his Body and Blood in the form of bread and wine. We Catholics believe that during the mass, these elements are changed forever and are the food from heaven. In consuming the Body and Blood of Jesus, he becomes closer to us than anyone ever could.

I was distracted on this day; I led the shortest Eucharistic prayer just trying to make it through. I especially had a tough time gripping the tiny flat round hosts in my hands that are the Body of Jesus. I was supposed to distribute them to the people.

"I can take care of this, Father. You seem to be struggling," said the kind woman who read our scriptures that day. I can't imagine what was going through her head when she saw me, but she instinctively took care of me. I sat down and prayed silently for my future asking Jesus to give me strength to get through. I wondered if it is just rest I needed. I would be okay, right?

After mass I touched base with the parish administrative assistant, AnnMarie, who said, "You look wiped Fr. Barrett."

"My hands and feet are tingling."

"You need to see a doctor. We need you to stay healthy."

"All right. I suppose I should go."

She was wise and usually spot on. I did fit in a meeting before taking time to get to the doctor. I ended up driving myself to Urgent Care at Park Nicolette in Burnsville, feeling overwhelmed as I went up to the desk.

"What seems to be the problem?" asked the receptionist in her forties with curly hair who hardly looked up from her computer.

"I'm not really sure, I have tingling in my hands and feet. I also feel woozy all over."

She now looked at me with much more compassion and told me to have a seat. I moved to some blue industrial-looking chairs to wait my turn. In my own little world of self-pity, I couldn't focus on anyone else. My stomach growled as I failed to eat lunch that day.

After what felt like an eternity, a pleasant young nurse called me back and took my vitals. She tried to make small talk, but I was pretty self-absorbed. After another long wait, I saw a male doctor probably a little younger than me. I repeated my symptoms. He said, "Have you been sick for a long time?"

"No, it came on yesterday. I'm so tired from my car trip to Nashville."

"I don't know how that would relate to this."

He had a bewildered look on his face and was slumping. I thought he was confused. The smartest thing he did was when he told me to see my doctor. My regular physician was busy, so they scheduled me with a Park Nicolet internist the next day, who was in the same building as the Urgent Care. I was frustrated and tired after the appointment and headed home.

Friday was my day off. I got up late around eleven, threw on some loose-fitting clothes and headed outside. It almost felt like a wall-banging hangover with my hands and feet like lead weights. The bright sun felt good on my skin. I took it easy and made it to my 1:00 appointment with the internist. She, like the Urgent Care doctor, seemed stumped with what was wrong with me. The petite woman in her forties said in what seemed like frustration. "So you're not sure how you got these symptoms?" I shook my head and she went on, "It could be neurological, stress-related, or something else. A few of your symptoms match something like cardiac or endocrinology. We are going to have to test you for many things." She was writing rapidly, not looking at me when she spoke.

The woman at the front desk was so kind. We scheduled the tests in the next couple of weeks and one was about a month out. They included a neurology exam, a cardiology stress test, and a colonoscopy. There might have been another one, too, but things were a blur. I left the doctor's office totally overwhelmed.

Then I drove the short trip from my doctor's office in Burnsville to the fairgrounds in Farmington to join my family. I had some bonding time with my family. My parents, brothers and their wives were around, but my attention was on my nephew Peter. He was a blonde-haired, blue-eye, strong, little guy, who loved all things sports. He was eight and was already quite a baseball player.

"Are you still playing ball, Peter?"

"Done for now until fall ball. Can I have one of those candy sticks?" He points to a brightly colored candies in old time jars at the mock general store we were near. The store is part of a heritage village from the late 1800s, which is one of the attractions at the fair. I looked to his mom, Melissa, who nodded and said, "You can have one, Peter."

I bought one for Peter and one for me. Mine was supposed to be watermelon, but the candy tasted awful. It had a metallic taste. Later I would realize that the illness was affecting my sense of taste. I noticed this taste in my sloppy gyro. I got cucumber sauce everywhere. My strawberry malt was also pretty disgusting.

The temperature was warm out, and a group of my family members saved seats for the *Arts In*. This was a musical put on by 4H youth that included my niece Tiana. Seeing the *Arts In* was a tradition, and it was more special with "T" in it. I felt woozy all over at the performance.

I walked with difficulty. I was so lucky that my brother Ed was on the fair board. He gave me a lift in his personal golf cart. I was so proud of him for he is ten years younger than me and has accomplished so much. I struggled to find my car and was embarrassed about that. This doesn't seem to bother Ed as we actually had a good laugh about it. He patiently drove me down the rows until we spied my bright blue Ford Focus. I liked my little car, and I was thrilled to see it. Also, I was grateful for Ed's help.

I remembered being just so tired. That journey home was a living odyssey, but I thought I could do it. I pulled out of the parking lot of the fairgrounds and tried to focus on my driving. Maneuvering seemed impossible to negotiate the grounds, but I managed to not hit any pedestrians. The main road worried me as I tried to keep the car between the lines. I took the State Highway first. When I got to the county road, which I knew well, I relaxed. The trip usually took me about forty minutes, but I was going to take it slow. My hands trembled on the steering wheel. I struggled for control. My feet tingled and felt like lead weights. I kept a close eye on my speed as I wasn't sure what I would say if I got pulled over. I knew I probably shouldn't be behind the wheel. My mind was racing, and I was just plain scared. What was happening to me? Why was it happening to me? I just wanted to get home safe and not be a threat to others.

As I headed west, I thought that I should have talked one of my brothers into driving me home. But they were so busy that I didn't want to be a burden. After all, when I was ordained a priest, I chose a life with a great deal of alone time.

I was almost home. Taking the county road right into town, I would negotiate a few streets in the town of Montgomery. I knew them well, but I struggled to keep the car on the right side of the street. Finally I made it to my garage after the wild ride, but the turmoil was continuing. I braced myself as I tried to get out of the car and found getting out a real struggle. It was like trying to get out of a seat of a carnival ride. The only difference was, things kept spinning. I felt drunk or drugged without having taken anything. I wondered how I would operate my numb and tingling fingers to lock the garage and to open the house door. Once inside, the steps to my room took maximum effort, and I rested several times before reaching the top. I almost fell as I entered my set of rooms on the upper floor. The rooms were an absolute mess. Papers, books, pizza boxes, a dead plant, and a whole host of other pathetic stuff in my mountain of a mess. I vow to clean, but this vow wouldn't materialize anytime soon. I got ready for bed. I took breaks and concentrated on my failing fingers. I finally collapsed into my bed. I knew I would fall right to sleep as I was wiped out.

I didn't set an alarm, figuring I could sleep in and still finish my weekend homily. I wasn't due at Pioneer Power until the afternoon. This is an antique grounds that was home to a little village and a place for old-time tractors. I had to be there by 4:00 p.m. to see the dedication of one of our churches that had been moved there. I was also be scheduled for the 8:15 p.m. mass at St. Scholastica. I was a mess now, but surely sleep would help.

Chapter 3

I've Fallen Twice

"Yet it was our infirmities he bore, our suffering he endured while we thought of him as stricken as he was smitten by God and afflicted." (Isaiah 53:4)

My eyes opened to a fuzzy world without the use of my glasses. I squinted to see my alarm clock. Wow, it was already 10:30 in the morning. I felt horrible, like I'd been hit by the proverbial truck. The shades were drawn, but the midmorning sun had tried to peek in. I had an excruciating pain in my feet, legs, and hands that felt like hundreds of tiny, hot needles poking away at me. It was a violent tingle and far more intense than yesterday. My arms and legs felt weighed down with lead. They were tough to move, so I continued to lay prone in my bed. I had a throbbing pain in my head. There was a deep ache in my back like when it acts up from time to time. I felt so many diverse types of pains. I had my own symphony of pain.

The room was warm, as if I had a little heater that had run unnecessarily on this August day. With the windows closed, the air was a bit stale. There was a big laundry pile in the open hamper and some of the clothes smelled pungent of sweat. A huge stack of books wobbled too close to the edge of the nightstand. They were unread books mostly, ranging from mystery to theology.

As I stared at this hoarded junk, I wondered if I tolerated this little disorder to keep the creative juices flowing. I might have just been lazy and disorganized. Even with the deep throbs of pain, I looked over the heaped mess and thought it was getting really bad and I needed to clean up.

As I struggled to sit up, I felt a needle-like pain ripping into my limbs. I placed my feet on the floor, and I attempted to rise. I fell to the ground with a big crash, and I landed on my stomach. After the initial shock, I crawled a bit and then attempted to get up again. This time I tried to use my dresser. But I put so much weight on it that both the dresser and I collapsed like a building going through demolition. The pain was like I took a large hit from a bulldozer. I lie there stunned with this very large piece of furniture on top of me. I was filled with a mind-numbing pain that spiked to new horizons as I struggled to get out from under the dresser. My pain was small compared to what Jesus must have felt, but for a brief moment I found some union with him. Now what was I to do? The pain and tingling were spiking in my hands and feet. It took maximum effort, but eventually I worked my way out from under the dresser.

At first I felt relief, but then my mind started to panic because I wasn't sure what to do next. After two falls, I realized something was horribly wrong. I racked my brain and wondered what to do. I felt too weak to yell, and the other priests might not have been in their rooms anyway. After all it was late morning.

Finally, I remembered that my phone was on my night-stand. I found it hard to move my hands and my feet, but somehow I crawled over there. I nervously held my phone and found it difficult to dial 911. I urged my fingers on as I struggled with this simple task. There was the 9, and it hurt when I pushed down with an extra throb. Despite the pain, I worked through it and pressed the 1 key twice. I was relieved that my call went through.

"911, how can I help you?"

"I've fallen twice, and my legs don't seem to work."

Stay on the line, and we will get someone there right away." The woman said with reassurance. I described where I was, and she comforted me as I gave her infor-mation. I'm not really sure what I told her. It seemed like forever before they got here. Hammering pain con-tinued to roll over me.

Later, I found out that the ambulance workers strug-gled to get into the strange structure I lived in. The rec-tory consisted of a basement and two floors with many rooms. All had mostly closed doors. I decided to crawl from my bedroom to my sitting room so they would have less trouble finding me. There were a number of pieces of furniture in this room, but there was a large open space in the middle of the room easily accessible through the door that led to the hallway. The room was always a bit untidy, but near my couch there was a suitcase from the car trip to Nashville I got back from a week ago that made it look messy. The clothes were out of the suitcase, but gifts and toiletries were sprawled out around it. I had been going nonstop until the last couple of days brought me to grinding halt.

I heard a knock at the door and was overcome with relief. I called out, and the door came open to reveal two paramedics. One was a tall stocky man and the other was a much shorter, petite woman who right away seemed to be in charge. They immediately stooped down and worked on me. Gently the woman took my vitals, and they got me on a gurney. Her voice was soothing, and I remembered the tone calmed me for a brief moment. She seemed familiar, but I didn't put it together until seven months later, when I visited with her at a party and my vague memories came back. She said that it was pretty weird knowing the person she was helping. She said that this didn't happen very often, and that it was surprising.

She asked a series of questions like, "Fr. Dave, where does it hurt?"

"All over."

"When did the pain start?"

"Wednesday."

"Do you know what caused the pain?"

"I have no idea." I said, growing weary of the questions. There were a ton of probing questions that bothered me at the time, but now I know they were just trying their best to care for me. In the frustration, I offered it up to God. I found some comfort in the chaos because I knew God was with me.

I looked around and realized a group of youth and adults were in my room. I learned later that they had been painting the new youth room in the basement and had let the paramedics in. They also had assisted in finding my room. Two of the leaders I knew well, Chris and Monica, had stooped down to pray with me. "We are here for you, Father" said Chris, who had short-cropped hair and a huge smile.

Monica said a prayer, "God, be with Father; help him not to be scared. Protect him from evil and help heal him. Amen."

I softly said, "Thank you."

Next, I remembered being lifted up and carried through the rectory as I watched the ceiling pass by. The straps provided a feeling of safety as I was carried down the steps that never seemed to end. I had walked them many times, but it is far different being carried down them.

I closed my eyes, wanting this adventure to end, but the pain kept burning inside of me. Even though things were looking pretty grim, I knew that somehow I was going to pull through. There were comforting voices

and steady hands that guided me into the ambulance
for the start of a monumental journey

Chapter 4

Local Hospital Does Good

"The Spirit of the Lord is upon me, because the Lord has anointed me . . ." (Isaiah 61:1)

A s we started out for the hospital, the intensity of my pain rose with every bump we went over. We were making a trip from Montgomery to New Prague, a trip I have made hundreds of times over the years. This was my first time riding in the back of an ambulance, and I knew I didn't want to make this a regular occurrence; in fact, even one more time would be too many. I don't recall lights or sirens, but I know I was distracted by the four-alarm fire of pain I was feeling throughout my poor body. The male paramedic was driving as we moved along and was talking with the female paramedic, who was working on me. Once in a while they asked me a question, but I wasn't very with it; my nemesis pain was getting in the way. I imagined myself on some TV show as we sped over the bumps, and this frightened me.

We finally made it to the emergency room of the Mayo Health Care Hospital in New Prague. I had visited patients here many times before. I even ministered a few times in the ER. This time was very different. Now I was the patient, and that thought frightened me as they

20

rolled me in. I was a shocked by the bright lights of the hospital. They rolled me through the doors and into a curtained-off room. I lay with all my worried thoughts and said a simple prayer of "Come, Lord Jesus," hoping that God would get me though this.

The nurse said, "Where is your pain, Father?"

"Hands and feet, but really all over."

"On a scale of one to ten, how would you rate your pain?"

"Eight . . . I don't know . . . Nine?"

I was having trouble focusing. She gave me a kind smile and said, "Hang in there, Father. The doctor will be here soon."

After a while I got to see a doctor. In a professional, yet caring voice, he said to me. "Hello Father. The EMTs and nurses gave me your background. You have had tingling in your hands and feet for a few days and now you are experiencing paralysis in your legs. Is that about right?"

"Yes doctor, there's pain in my feet and legs as well."

He stood over six feet tall and had the look of someone who really knew his way around the ER. He wore a long white lab coat with dark hair and a well-weathered face that made me think he was a few years older than me. He looked me right in the eyes and said, "From what you are telling me, I believe you may have Guillain Barré syndrome."

I had heard of this illness before, and I knew people didn't usually die from GBS. For a brief moment, the pain seemed to lessen, and some relief swept over me. Fr. Michael Joncus, a priest of the Archdiocese, who also was a composer, had GBS. There was also a patient I once saw when I was a hospital chaplain, who had this condition. I knew they had long, hard illnesses, but I also knew that they both got better.

The doctor went on. "Sorry to say, Father, things are probably going to get worse before they get better. People usually come out of it pretty well, but it's a long road."

"It's not normally fatal, right?"

"That's right, but you will have to be closely monitored. I hear you want to go to Methodist, right?"

"Yes, I belong to Park Nicollet health system. My sister works for Park Nicollet, and the hospital is fairly close to where she lives."

I didn't know what would lay ahead, but I knew I could beat it. I was going to be sick, but I knew God wanted me to live. Even though that gave me some consolation, I was still torn up with pain and wished I didn't have to go through with the long haul that laid before me.

I'm not sure who it was, but someone asked me if I wanted to call a loved one, and a nurse gave me my phone. There was some pain in my hand from dialing the phone, but I called my dad's cell. He always seemed to know what to do. I also remembered that many in my family would be with him at the Dakota County Fair. I had been there last night. I tapped "send," and on the third ring, he picked up, "Hello, Dad?"

"No, Dave, it's Carol. I answered his phone because he is putting mustard on a corndog."

"Carol, I'm really sick in the hospital in New Prague, and they are going to send me to Methodist."

"Here's Joan." She said with a scared tone in her voice. She was always a bit squeamish when it came to hospitals. I'm sure I just shocked her.

"Hello, Dave, what about Methodist Hospital?"

It was my sister, Joan, the medical social worker. She was the steady one who knew what to do in emergency situations. I gathered myself and said, "I have tingling in my hands and feet and paralysis in my legs. I'm in New Prague, but I'm transferring to Methodist soon."

"Don't worry Dave, it won't take us long to get there. Try to stay calm, and we will meet you there."

"Thanks, Joan." I felt reassured she would be there to support me. With that, the call ended.

Fr. Kevin Clinton, my boss, and Deacon Bob Wagner, my trusty co-worker, came and visited me. Kevin asked me if he could anoint me with the sacrament of the sick. I agreed. Having been a former hospital chaplain, I had anointed people hundreds of times, and now it was happening to me. Some people believed anointing was only meant for the dying. The Church has been trying to broaden its use and take it back to earlier origins, using it for any stage of illness. The onset of my GBS was the perfect time, and Kevin knew this when he offered me the sacrament that I was overjoyed to receive.

He made the sign of the cross when he touched his forehead, his heart, and both shoulders and said, "In the name of the Father and of the Son and of the Holy Spirit"

"Amen," we said together. Deacon Bob and I made the same gestures in silence with Fr. Kevin. He continued, "As it was said by the Apostle James, 'are there any sick among you? If there are let us send for the priests of the Church and the priests can anoint them with the oil of salvation. The oil will save the sick person and if they have committed any sins may their sins be forgiven.'"

Fr. Kevin then prayed a simple prayer. Deacon Bob and I said, "Amen."

When Fr. Kevin placed his hands on my head and prayed in silence, his hands felt very warm as the heat extended from his hands like the Holy Spirit. Deacon Bob also prayed as he placed his hand on my shoulder. My tense shoulders started to relax, and I, too, prayed for healing and endurance. Then Fr. Kevin opened a small container of oil and wet his thumb in it. He traced the sign of the cross on my forehead while saying, "Through this holy anointing, may God give you the grace of the Holy Spirit." As he put more oil on his thumb and made crosses on each of my hands, he said, "May the God who frees you from sin save you and raise you up."

The oil soaked into my skin, infusing God's healing mercies within me. I was overwhelmed with gratitude and felt a sense of being protected. The three of us prayed the Our Father prayer and Fr. Kevin blessed me. "I bless you in the name of the Father and of the Son and of the Holy Spirit."

I was glad Deacon Bob was there. He and I shared a great deal during his illness. He had a hip replacement which became infected for the better part of ten months. I remember thinking it was so nice to be with the clergy I worked with for this anointing, which has already starting to calm my spirit. Fr. Kevin and Deacon Bob would be instrumental in covering the ministry of my churches in my absence. While we visited, they assured me things would be fine. We talked until a nurse came and told me they were ready to transfer me to Methodist.

I don't remember a lot about the trip from Mayo in New Prague to Methodist in St. Louis Park. I remembered praying that God would not forsake me. Things would be okay, right? I tried to remind myself that I wasn't in control; God was.

Chapter 5

Joan and the ICU

"Who can come into your presence as vindicator of unjust men?" (Wisdom 12:12c)

My memory of most of my Methodist Hospital stay was a blur. I was in and out like a far-off radio station, and some of the time I was in an induced coma. My sister Joan told me that this was a blessing. Joan is eleven years younger than me, but we have always been close. I have rejoiced in what a fine woman she has become. Joan is very bright and the type of person you want on your side. She has a bit of an artistic talent. When she was in college, she gave me a hand-painted frame with a picture of us. The frame said, "Not only a brother, but a friend." I admired Joan for her solid marriage to Tim, and she is a great mom to her son, Andrew, my nephew and God child. She cared deeply for all the members of our family and had at times been a help to us all.

I believed I was a support for her when she was growing up. I babysat her countless times, organized work crews for her to help on the farm, and coached her softball teams. One time, I remember I talked with her about a boyfriend she had been concerned about because he didn't practice his faith. Now she has returned the favor to be my medical advocate. This was made easier by her role as a medical social worker for Park Nicollet's Struthers Parkinson Center.

I also relied on my sister to help me with my memory. It felt so weird to have a blur in my life, not be able to readily recall ten days of my life. I have been told by a number of sources that I was out of it much of the time and panicked quite a bit of my waking time. This was uncomfortable. For most of the rest of my life, I have been conscious and in charge of my circumstances unless I was asleep.

A little over a year after my hospitalization, Joan and I sat down together, and I tried to piece the events together. Joan at the time was in her mid-thirties and was a take-charge person, yet she was extremely likable. As we talked, Joan looked at me with her kind green eyes on this cold autumn night.

We sat in her basement at the nice wooden bar complete with Michelob Golden light draft on tap. She had a beer. I settled on a water because of the medication I was taking. We turned toward each other as she told me about those early days. "After you had called us during our Dakota County Fair visit, Carol, Nick, and I along with Mom and Dad came to the hospital just after you got there. They had admitted you into neurology right from the emergency room. We walked into the room when a doctor was giving you neurology screening tests. He would tell you to lift your arm or your leg, and you couldn't. He would ask you to feel taps he made on your arms and legs with a small hammer. You couldn't do that, either."

Joan was shaking as she relayed this. There was fear in her bright-green eyes. I was hanging on her every word. I had heard parts of this story before, but this was in much more detail. I took a sip from my glass with my feet glued to the rung of the padded bar stool. I asked a quick question. "Were you scared for me?"

"Very much so. You were pretty out of it. You were responding to the doctor, but you looked so tired, almost numb. It was in this moment that I realized just how sick you were."

"Wow, I don't remember this."

"Probably for your own protection" she replied with a caring voice. "Despite the assurance the New Prague doctor gave you about the diagnosis of GBS, the doctor at Methodist wasn't so sure. In his mind, there wasn't enough background information to justify this rare disease.

"Right, I hadn't just gotten a flu or any other vaccine or I hadn't gone through a long flu-like illness, both of which would have linked me more to GBS."

"GBS was usually carried by a virus. He would have to run more tests to be sure."

"He didn't start the treatments right away?"

"No, because of his caution, the blood treatment didn't begin right away." Joan said.

I was shaking a bit, thinking of how my loved ones saw me at such a low point. I felt especially sad for my parents. Joan with a steady voice continued. "The family was really freaking out. Carol took it especially hard. You remember how she was with Grandma and Sophie. She was a little better now that she's older, but it was still very hard on her."

Carol is the baby of our family, now in her early thirties. In high school, she had a terrible time with the death of my mom's mom and Grandma's sister. She would end up being very sweet and caring during my recovery process but struggled at first. She and her husband, Nick, had only been married a few months, and he was a great comfort to her. We had interacted quite a bit around the time of the wedding as I had the Mass. Nick and I often chatted at family gatherings, and I really enjoyed him as part of our family. I considered myself fairly close to Carol, who was fourteen years younger than me. Without Carol, I don't know if I would have survived this illness.

"How were Mom and Dad?" I said.

"Quiet, but strong, and they let me be in charge."

Dad was a farmer who, at seventy-three, was very strong with the resiliency of a much younger man. He wasn't perfect, but as I matured, I started to accept him for who he is. My mom is a retired farm worker, school cook, and grocery store cashier. She still keeps the farm books and enjoys life as a full-time grandma. She is a young seventy-one, who enjoys water aerobics and outings with her friends. My parents are people of faith who were to be with me no matter what. Oftentimes a priest develops a special relationship with his parents. I enjoy spending time with them, and I try to see them often. I don't let a week go by without calling them.

Joan told me that my family finally started to realize just how sick I was. I was only in neurology for a short time before they brought me to ICU. I rapidly went down from there. Even though my parents knew I had some symptoms from the day before, they weren't prepared for this. They had the opportunity to see me in my ICU room and get a little information about the testing that was done there. Mostly, the doctors and nurses would see how I progressed during my hospital stay. I guess I sort of stabilized, and everyone went home on Saturday night.

My sisters and their husbands came on Sunday. It was a fairly uneventful day, while they mainly monitored me, but gradually over time my condition continued to worsen. Joan said she went home that night and started my CaringBridge site. This interactive Internet site proved to be a valuable link between my family and the many people who cared for and prayed for me. I was told that different people read the tributes and commented to me through the early part of my hospital stay. I read them later, and I really enjoyed all of the comments and tributes, but I somehow didn't believe that I deserved this much love. One tribute really stuck

out. It described me as "a humble man of simple faith."
I vowed to try and live out this observation every day
of my life.

Joan took a sip of her beer and went on, "Monday
proved to be a real bad day. You could no longer breathe
on you own and were put on a ventilator." I had seen a
number of people on ventilators and had been shaken by
the experience. A nurse who worked in an ICU, whose
child I baptized, told me that being on the vent was
never very fun for anyone. She said the ventilator was
violent to the body.

Joan told me that they put me on heavy sedation to mit-
igate the stress from the ventilator. Most of the family
was there that night, including my four siblings. Joan
wanted them to take shifts to watch me so that someone
would be there when doctors visited. They also would
be able to brief visitors about what was going on. She
was annoyed that this suggestion was met with a little
resistance. My brother Rich gave staying with me a
try, but watching me made him feel helpless. He was a
problem solver, and I was a problem that didn't have an
immediate solution. My brother Ed, three years younger
than Rich, was pretty busy during the time of my illness,
which was why he often sent his wife Kayla. I think Ed
was also a bit freaked out by hospitals.

Joan took many shifts, taking some time off work to be
with me. She said, "I would often work part of the day
and then try and work from my laptop in your room."

"Could you get anything done?" I asked. I was starting to feel guilty about all the time she spent with me.

"It was hard to work because there were so many people in and out of an ICU room. I was so blessed that I had such a caring workplace."

"Sounds like you dealt with it well."

She nodded and smiled and went on to tell me that there were two ICU neurologists who came around during my stay. One was a woman who came the most, and Joan found her quite helpful. She did a good job of explaining things to the family. She really respected Joan as my advocate as a medical social worker. This doctor was thorough, and I believe helped me a great deal.

The other doctor was a man who had a thick, foreign accent. She couldn't tell what country he was from. Joan found this man less than agreeable. One particular day came when they decided to try and lower my sedation so they could get me off the vent and out of the ICU. I was having a bad day, saying things that were impossible like having been in a pool downstairs and that I got to take a shower. Joan and a nurse tried to reason with me. They assured me that there wasn't a pool on a lower floor and that this room didn't have a shower. Evidently I wasn't buying it. They made a little headway when a male nurse came and told me I was suffering from hallucinations, a common problem among ICU patients, and I should try and calm down. His effort was only partially effective, but Joan knew those outbursts were not normal for me. I was off my medication, but Joan thought that a little Ativan would help. The nurse needed the doctor's approval to administer the drug. The doctor was coming to my room next.

When this doctor and the intern got to my room, they stayed in the hallway and spoke in hushed tones. The woman doctor had always come into the room and involved Joan in the conversation. Joan overheard that they wanted to use a drug called Haldol instead of Ativan because Ativan would perhaps slow down the time it took to come off the vent. Joan interjected herself into their conversation because she knew Haldol was a very heavy-duty antipsychotic. She had known from experience that if using Haldol was in my chart, every doctor would simply go to this drug, and it would basically knock me out. Joan didn't think I needed this and argued for the Ativan, which I would use frequently from then on. The doctor at first wondered how she knew all those drug names. The intern pointed out that Joan was a medical social worker, who was my sister and had followed my hospital stay from the beginning.

As Joan spoke of the doctor, she started to tap her beer glass. I heard her voice crack and saw the tension in her face as she explained the argument. "After much back and forth with raised voices; the doctor finally allowed Ativan and that did the trick." She said triumphantly.

Joan told me she was a wreck from defending me and not having enough sleep. When she left the room, she saw that Mom and Dad came up the hallway, and she burst into tears when she reached them. She told me that she wasn't going to let that doctor see her cry. After relaxing in the family lounge for a while, Mom slipped down to the hospital gift shop and bought her a scarf. Joan wore that scarf like a medal; she was my champion.

Chapter 6

Tim and the Bad Dream

"Such was his intention when behold, the angel of the Lord appeared to him in a dream and said, 'Joseph, Son of David, do not be afraid'" (Matthew 1:20).

> "Twin's drop another to the Sox. The Twins look feeble as they give up another game to visiting Chicago. The deficiencies on the mound are only equal to the three errors on defense."

Tim, my brother-in-law, reported these headlines. All of a sudden, I found myself in a dream. I'm not sure if it was drug induced or if I was so tired that I was going in and out of consciousness.

My dream put me on a video screen. I looked at myself in a mirror. I was a cartoon character with huge exaggerated facial features. I wore a checked kelly-green shirt, blue pants, and sunshine yellow shoes, all of which glowed.

> "It's only mid-August and the Twins are literally playing out the schedule."

I was at the start of a red maze. I saw a huge black monster that stood at least seven feet tall with three long arms and chubby legs next to the entrance. He was slow-moving, fat, and hairy. He seemed to weigh over 400 pounds. He had red beady eyes with blue smoke coming out of the mouth of his deranged black-skinned face. The monster moved toward me, threatening me with his long arms and grunts. I was forced to run into the maze to avoid him. Brown vines that lay on the path grabbed my feet and my legs, causing me to trip. The creature on his part lumbered after me and I just kept running.

> "Let's see about the Vikings. It says here
> that Christian Ponder has looked good in
> limited practice during training camp."

I kept running, but I glanced over my shoulder to see the monster gaining on me. I ran into the moss-covered walls and doubled back. The vines popped up and twisted around my feet. I broke free and made a right turn in the maze, but I looked back and the monster just kept coming. Hot smoke singed my back, and the smell of sulfur was in the air. I heard the monster breathing hard and the loud pounding of his feet as they clomped around the maze.

> "The Gophers are looking sharp in prac-
> tice as they prepare to open up against
> Middle Tennessee State at the Bank on
> Saturday night. Hey I think Nick and
> Carol are going to the game."

I saw a straight way that had very few vines. I sped to get away from the monster. I felt pretty good, and I looked for ways to get out of the head-high maze. I tried to see over the top, but all I saw was more maze in every direction. I just kept running.

> "How about some CaringBridge? Here's
> one from a Fr. Stan, 'Dave I hope you
> heal soon. I know you will survive.'"

I felt relief as the monster was far behind. I ran until I reached a dead end. I jumped up, trying to get out of the maze, but it got much taller, and I couldn't reach the top. The monster just kept coming, and I couldn't go anywhere because I was backed into a corner. I really start to panic as it looked as if the beast was going to get me. I took one final jump and went over the maze. Things faded to black.

Throughout the reading, Tim's voice had grown fainter and fainter like I was running away from him. I was terrified. His voice was comforting, but soon it became so faint that I drifted off into nothingness. This dream that competed with my brother-in-law haunted me for a long time. I prayed about it, and eventually I made some sense out of what was a vivid and scary dream. I found bright colors pleasing to the eye, so I had my room painted orange when I was in high school. I wanted it really bright, but my parents asked me to tone it down a bit, and I reluctantly agreed.

Green has always been an important color. I love the bright kelly green like the fields I saw in Ireland. I also have a love-hate relationship with green. When I was in junior high, one of the bullies on my bus dumped green paint all over me after I got off the bus. He dumped it out the window and hit me when the back of the bus swung around while I went to check for mail. I was covered in green paint, and everyone on the bus roared with laughter. I had to march up the hill to my house in tears to face my mother. She helped me clean up. It was tempera paint, so it washed off easily, and at least I was home when it happened.

I believe the monster represented GBS and all of my fears. Even though part of me knew that the chances of my recovery were that high, I still had fear. This fear was so captivating. I had a disease that scared the living daylights out of me, and I felt powerless. I knew most people recovered from GBS, but when and how made me scared. So I ran!

In days when I was younger and weighed less, I ran long distances. I ran the 5K event in junior college and ran a few more of those races in my late twenties. Running was an escape for me, and I would probably still be running if I hadn't gotten so heavy over the years. So, for me to run was common in many of my dreams. I ran while being chased by all problems that affected me.

Fear seemed pretty evil, and this made me wonder if I still suffered from shame or had feelings of not being forgiven. I had done things that I wasn't proud of. I had hurt others and done some devastating things to my self-worth. I was in a state where I thought God wouldn't forgive me, even though I had been told this was not logical. I had gone to reconciliation many times, but it never seemed to stick. Perhaps I was in this terrible state of mind because I couldn't forgive myself. This lead to a long loneliness that at times made me uncomfortable in my own skin.

I realized that the monster catching up to me in the corner was significant. Was I going to become totally overwhelmed or even die? Was the monster going to catch me? As I thought about it more, my last action was jumping out of the maze. In my younger days, I was a part-time jumper when I wasn't being a distance runner. In my dream, I seemingly jumped into recovery. The road ahead would be long, but I was in it for the long haul.

Chapter 7

Methodist Therapies

"If one loves justice the fruits of her works are virtues for she teaches moderation and prudence, justice and fortitude and nothing in life is more useful than these." (Wisdom 8:7)

The sickness was slowly leaving me. At this point I was starting to talk, but I was just too weak for people to understand me. Speech Therapist Karen was pure goodness. I was drawn to her, although I can't even remember what she looked like. I just know that she was good at her job, and I was making great strides under her tutelage. She was like a warm feeling one has when one smells hot apple pie. Joan told me that I liked her and seemed to look forward to her coming to give me therapy. I was still pretty out of it in those early days, so it was good to get the feedback from Joan.

Speech Therapist Karen would give me breathing exercises. "Okay Dave, let's try and get a big breath, for all speech begins with breath," she said. I wanted to please her, and I remember trying with all my might to get air into my lungs. "That's really good, Dave. Now try to make a la sound. Try la, la, la."

No sound came out, and I was disappointed.

"Try it again. Don't force it. Let the sounds flow out of you."

I took another deep breath and softly a few "la's" escaped my mouth. I was elated, and I realized this was a first step in getting my voice back.

"Great, Dave! That is what we're looking for. Let's repeat it, and I bet you will get better."

I breathed deeply again and tried to exhale all of the air out of my lungs. I was now tired, but I was driven. I let off another couple of "la's."

"Wow that was incredible. You are getting better and better. Dave, you will speaking before you know it," she said with enthusiasm.

I welled with pride; I knew I was getting better. With the help of God, I would speak again.

These exercises reminded me a bit of voice lessons I had in the seminary. Breathing was a big part of this. I would do exercises to build up my diaphragm. Here in the hospital I had to strengthen my body, so I could make sound again. I think the biggest obstacle I faced with my speech was being heard. This was rather ironic because a strong voice was one of my trademarks. I had been told that my voice was a bit overpowering for some. Most people, especially older people, really appreciated the booming voice I used in church. In my two small churches, I never used a microphone.

*****

Nurse Linda was setting up the blood-cleaning machine over my left shoulder. I couldn't see much, but I heard her working with both plastic and metal. There were some thumping and tinging sounds as she put this apparatus together. I thought of her like some kind of mad scientist, who volunteered to fight the disease, roaming within me.

"It won't take long to get you hooked up. This isn't a transfusion, and we won't be adding anyone else's blood into yours. We are just cleaning your blood and putting it back in there. It's a painless process that will take about three hours. We will have to repeat the process about three times. I will probably be the one treating you the whole time."

Plasmapheresis is the removal, treatment, and return of the components of blood plasma from blood circulation. It is a medical procedure performed outside the body. This type of filtering is the most common method used in GBS. This procedure may also help against Lupus.

"You can just relax, David, the machine will do all the work" said Nurse Linda with her soothing voice. I would fade in and out while Linda spent most of her time at the machine behind me. I remembered a reassuring humming noise that the machine made. It made sense that if the blood was tainted with GBS, which attacked the nerves, it would have to be removed. My body could then focus on healing, rather than fighting the disease. Healing was happening, yet I still lay paralyzed.

Nurse Linda was another valuable link in the chain of my healing. Many great people were in that chain. Many of the links at Methodist are unknown to me. It blows my mind to think that so many people would work on my behalf. I realized they were doing their jobs, but I am grateful. Healing is about connection and community. Disease breaks us apart, and we find ourselves separated. We feel alone in illness and are in need of reconnection. This couldn't be done on our own. One of the gifts of GBS is that I have learned how I can depend on others. I don't have to do everything myself. I can be made whole again by the help of others. The blood cleaning helped me physically, but the whole process of healing has shaped me mentally and spiritually as well. I'm so glad Nurse Linda was a part of my life.

*****

Sometimes therapy happens when we don't even realize it. During my time at Methodist, I had spiritual therapy in the form of intercessory prayer. Joan told me I got a message from my classmate, Fr. Michael Reding, who was pastor at St. Bartholomew's in Wayzata. He had always been like a big brother even though he is only about six months older. He wrote this inspiring message on my CaringBridge page when I was suffering in the ICU:

Fr. Dave,

Thanks to Fr. Don, the news of your illness was conveyed to your classmates quickly, and I know that we are all praying for you. Be assured also of the prayers of my parishioners at Saint Bartholomew, and know that I will offer mass for you next week. I know that GBS can be a long and difficult trial, but I also know that our merciful and compassionate God never leaves your side. As you experience your own Calvary, know that he accompanies you and that many of us stand at the foot of your cross, offering our prayers.

I recall that your favorite place in the Holy Land was the Church of All Nations in the Garden of Gethsemane. It appears now that the Lord will not "take this cup from you" immediately, but as with Christ in the Garden, you can be assured that he will send his angels to minister to you and strengthen you. Those angels include your family, your parishioners, and your brother priests. I pray that you feel our support.

You have much more to accomplish for the glory of God, so be strong.

Fr. Michael Reding

GBS was very much my Gethsemane where I was undergoing pain and trial. I asked God *Why?* I wanted to accept my suffering and move toward a solution. I wanted to follow God's will and drink the cup of His suffering. I knew it was God's will that I serve as a priest. Things looked bleak in my hospital room, but I knew that better days lay ahead. I loved that Fr. Michael referenced the Church of All Nations as it has always had special meaning for me.

Outside this special church, located on the Mount of Olives, there is a beautiful grove of olive trees. I loved to sit by those trees and reflect on what Jesus went through. Those trees were very old and were like the trees during the time of Jesus. The church had beautiful mosaics depicting Christ in the garden and various saints that I couldn't identify. The mosaics were high on the structure just below the roof line, and they were colorful in soft tones of red, yellow, and blue. The church was fairly plain on the inside, lots of stone and a few colorful windows. The lighting was dim, and there was a lingering scent of incense in the dry air. The most striking part was a black wrought-iron fence around a big, gray rock. This area is set off because it was treated like the place of the prayer, where Jesus accepted his suffering before his arrest. Jesus prayed while his closest followers slept just a few yards away.

As a seminarian in 1995, I spent a great deal of time in that church. I was given the opportunity to pray on that rock by the Franciscan priest in charge. It was emotional and moving to pray there at the probable spot where Jesus prayed 2,000 years ago. It blew my mind that I was at least close to where he prayed. The stone was hard and cold beneath me, but the pure emotion of being there overrode any discomfort. I prayed for my vocation and for all my loved ones. I prayed for the poor and the unemployed. I was also praying for peace in this region and in the whole world. I also just wanted to let God give me strength and courage to rest in his light.

I traveled there in 2007 as a priest with my classmates. We took turns presiding at mass at the various churches. As soon as I saw we were going to the Church of All Nations, I immediately signed up. I have a beautiful picture of myself in a red chasuble at that church. Three of my classmates are to my right, and three are to my left each dressed in a white alb and a red stole. Red is the color that represents the passion of Christ. That picture represents a very proud moment for me.

I have gone through many trials, including a minor mental illness that plagued the early years of my priesthood. I had a lot to overcome. It took therapy, medication, and prayer to come out of my illness. I still deal with it, but I am happy to say that the mental illness is in remission.

I was overwhelmed with joy to be able to preach about my mental illness, comparing my suffering to the sufferings of Christ. I know he suffered much worse, but I still feel united with him. It was extremely powerful for me to share this message of hope with my classmates that day at the Church of All Nations.

A couple of months into my illness, Fr. Michael took a group of pilgrims to the Holy Land. After he returned he wrote this on my CaringBridge page:

> Dave,
>
> I'm so glad to hear of your continued progress. You have been in my prayers each day.
>
> I've just returned from leading a pilgrimage group of thirty-five to the Holy Land. On the evening of October 22, we spent a Holy Hour praying at the Church of All Nations in the Garden of Gethsemane. As we began our prayer that evening, I told the group about your condition and also told them that this was your favorite place for prayer in Jerusalem. I asked them to pray for you as you continue to endure your own agony. Their intercession was palpable that night as we kept watch for one hour with Christ.
>
> May you continue to know healing and be increasingly strengthened in the Lord.
>
> Your classmate,
>
> Michael Reding

The pilgrims prayed in adoration. This was done by exposing the Blessed Sacrament, a flat round disk, in a holder called a monstrance. We believe this disk that we call a host is really the body of Jesus Christ. This monstrance is often an ornate gold place of display that stands about eighteen inches tall and was made to show how special the host is. Often the gold is like rays of the sun coming off the real presence of the Son of God. It was normally placed on the church's altar, the place the sacrifice of the mass happened. Catholics believe that the Blessed Sacrament has the same substance as Jesus and that a host, after consecration is truly the Body of Jesus. Prayer before the Body of Christ is considered very powerful. I was powerless and their prayer, even though I didn't know them personally, gave me power. We were connected by faith, and their fervent prayer was spiritual help to me.

There were so many families and churches that were praying for me on a regular basis. It felt good to be constantly enveloped in communion with God. My family would mention the different people who were taking time to pray for me. God led me through the odyssey of my illness, but the road was lit by a pathway of prayer.

Chapter 8

Internal Struggles

"My God, my God, why have you forsaken me?"
(Matthew 27:46)

> Most of the time I felt like I was in a
> dream state. I couldn't tell minutes from
> days. There was no way to know if it
> was night or day. I heard loved ones
> talking, picked up snippets of conver-
> sation, without really putting things
> together. They usually weren't talking
> to me but about me. I didn't have my
> glasses on, so everything was a bit hard
> to see and added to my internal foggi-
> ness. My thoughts were often scattered,
> moving in many different directions.

After the Blue Angel experience, my brain would
play with the predicament of not being able to
move. This mental gymnastics was an internal struggle.
In the hospital, I had many dreams. I think they were
probably drug induced, but they were vivid to me,
and they carried immense meaning. Here is one of
the visions:

I was to be in a production of *The Lion King*. The nurse came in carrying a costume for me to wear. The costume looked fury and was rust colored. She smiled at me and said. "Here is your costume for the play; you are going to be a lion. Put it on and wait to be called."

She turned on the television to the hospital channel to show a stage. There was a loud booming voice coming from the television that said he was the director. This man, who had a French accent, called out from the television for each patient to come forward. The screen showed a stage with many actors dressed in natural colors of brown, avocado green, tan, and rust. They were responding to the different stage directions given by the voice.

The nurse said "He is a world-renowned director, and we are lucky to have him. The stage is two floors down. It's really easy to find." I remember being nervous yet excited. She continued as I just lay there, unable to speak. "You will be great. Most patients have a lot of fun. The proceeds of the play help fund the hospital. All patients are encouraged to participate." With that she left the room.

I tried to get up to put my costume on, but my arms and legs didn't move. I lay there helpless. I tried to call out, but I had no voice. I didn't think she could hear me, anyway, since the door was shut. The director kept calling names. As each name was called, I worried about having my name called. I was afraid I was going to let down the production, and I got more anxious by the minute. Finally he called my name. He waited a little while and called it again. I felt overwhelmed and thought I had failed. I knew I would not be able to be in the production under my own power. I would need help putting on the lion costume. I would need help getting out of bed and getting into a wheelchair. I would need someone to wheel me down to the stage. I would even need to be put on stage. I would not be able to take direction without someone's help. I was in a state of total dependence.

This dream had a big impact on me. My helplessness was not a comforting thought. This fear made me really nervous because I wasn't always the best at trusting. I usually wanted to be my own man, to run my own show. This was not the case in my dream nor was this true in my GBS journey. So I thought about the mercy I needed from both God and the people in my life.

I thought about the significance of the production of *The Lion King*. I never saw it as a play in person, but I caught part of it on TV once. I also saw the movie a few times from my days of volunteering at the pediatric epilepsy wing of United Hospital in St. Paul. *The Lion King* was a favorite to most of the children. It had a great story of discovery for the young lion to evolve into a great king.

I have a friend who really likes all lions. He is particularly drawn to the image of the lion that lies down with the lamb from the eleventh chapter of the book of the prophet Isaiah. For me the image of the lion was more alive when Jesus was referred to in the book of Revelation as the Lion of Judah. I see this lion as strong and powerful. So, to put on my costume was to literally put on Christ.

I wanted to have faith, but the devil put so much fear in the way. What was the basis of that fear? I'm not sure, but I think it had to do with some doubts of my ability to be a good priest. Before I got sick, I wondered about how much I was needed. I certainly felt very much called to be a priest. I was pretty sure this is where God wanted me to be, but I wasn't sure I was using my gifts to the best of my abilities. I tried hard, but was that enough? I was now sick, and I knew I couldn't do things alone.

I was in a constant state of worry with questions whirling around in my head. Would I be able to move again, or was God getting me ready to lead a life where I was paralyzed? Would I be any good at moving around in a wheelchair? Would I still live in Montgomery and work in the New Prague area at my country churches? Would my voice return to preach, and would I have anything to say? Would I be able to consecrate the Eucharist or would the Body and Blood of Jesus ever enter my mouth again? I would try to formulate answers in my head, and they would lead to another question and then to moments of despair.

One of the ways I coped with the fear was relying on my family. I had a great family, and they were more support than I could ever ask for: loving parents, stalwart brothers, and the most loyal and supportive sisters a guy could ever ask for. Without being able to comprehend everything that was happening, I knew they were pulling for me. Like a dependable pair of shoes, I knew they would carry me through. They would walk me back to health.

In part of my mind, I knew I could count on the Holy Family as well. Joseph was called in a dream by the angels to be supportive of Mary and her divine son. Joseph would take the same care with me as he showed the Christ. Joseph represented the gentleness of a lily and the strength of a carpenter's square. The foster father of our Lord would help me along the way. I had the strength of the man who listened to his dreams and gained strength from solving problems that secured the safety of the boy Jesus. Decisions to go to Egypt and come back to Nazareth were timely because he was dependent upon and trusting God, the Heavenly Father.

Why should I have any doubts when I was in the care of a mother like Mary? She is the handmaid of the Lord, and I know she loves me, as well. Despite my human frailties, she has nothing but love for me. In her service, Mary is beautiful to behold. She cared for Jesus, yet she is also my spiritual mother. I felt her care in the many rosaries people prayed for me. Mary is the first disciple. She is the Church, and as her priest, I am loyal to the Church. Amidst the pain, I asked Mother Mary to pray for me.

Most of all I was cared for by the Holy Redeemer, Jesus Christ. He is both brother and Savior. He is the best friend I could ever have. Jesus is compassionate, meaning he suffers with me. GBS was my Calvary, and my pain was just a tiny portion of his cross. I was unable to do any of my formal prayer during my time at Methodist, but at times I was able to say in my mind the name Jesus, and this made all the difference. I have always had an affinity for the name of Jesus. It is why I end nearly every one of my homilies with, "the one who loved us first, that one being Jesus Christ." Over the years, I have thought about the meaning of those words. As a Christian, we are taught to love Jesus. We see him through scripture. I study scripture, and the wisdom of Jesus still amazes me, as much as when I first read about him in elementary school. But no matter how much I love him, the truth is that he loved me first.

Chapter 9

Cory and the Transfer to Neurology

"Pharaoh was already near when the Israelites looked up and saw the Egyptians were on the march in pursuit of them. In great fright they cried out to the Lord." (Exodus 14:10).

L ife for me in ICU was all about rest. As I came closer to getting out of ICU, I had more times of being awake. When I opened my eyes from one of my many naps, there was Cory. This was Fr. Cory Rolfing, who was about five years my junior and had been a priest four years less than I had been. It was so good to see him as he is a close brother-priest. We had served the parish in Montgomery together for four and a half years, and he was my landlord as I stayed living at the parish rectory in Montgomery even after my assignment switched to New Prague. I would say he was good looking, but modesty prevents it as people say we look so much alike. He is a little taller, my five feet, 9 inches to his just under six feet. We both wear our brown hair fairly short and both sport glasses with fairly similar frames. I had him by a few pounds, but neither of us are going to be confused with skinny. His skin was fairly tan, no doubt due to some extended time on the lake fishing. The tan skin was in contrast to the mostly white sterile atmosphere of my hospital room. I felt a slight whoosh of air as the humble priest entered my temporary home. Cory was easygoing, never getting too high or too low. We got well acquainted in that almost six years we spent under one roof. He was my boss, but he was always fair. Even when we didn't see things the same way, he still treated me with respect and compassion. I always tried to do the same with him.

"How are you feeling, David?"

"Not much at all," I gestured my head down to my lifeless hands and feet.

"You're not going to let a little thing like that get you down."

We both laughed along with my mom and dad, who I forgot were also in the room. "Thanks so much for coming to see him, Cory. I know it means a lot to Dave and to us," Mom said. They had met Cory a number of times over the years that I knew him, which went back a number of years before we worked together. "You liked working with Cory, didn't you Dave?" Mom said.

"Well, most of the time," I said.

"If he can jab at me, he must not be too sick," Cory said.

Cory gave me one of his mischievous smiles. For a few minutes, none of really talked as we were just enjoying each other's company without words. It was good to see a visitor—especially one like Cory who is so full of life. He is a good shepherd who serves his people well. He likes to fish, and now God has him fishing for all people. We talked about my progress, and we talked about prayer. I found myself with plenty of time for that.

A nurse walked in and said, "David, you got the okay to get out of ICU and into a room upstairs."

"You are moving up. I had better get going, and I will see you David," Cory said as he headed out.

I was excited about the move. It meant I was one step closer to going to a step-down hospital. Joan and I talked about the two options of Bethesda in St. Paul and Regency in Minneapolis. We had thought Regency would be a lot closer drive for Joan. Regency was also right next to Courage Center; the place where I really hoped to learn how to walk again.

All of this seemed to be moving too slow, but I knew God would slow me down, so I could learn the most from each situation I faced. Spiritually, I was still trusting in God, but I let the devil creep in every time things moved slower than I would like. I found out later that I was really progressing well, but when you're bed-ridden, it always seemed to slow. The devil was in the boredom and the doubt.

"Here come your movers" my dad said.

A man and a woman, both African American, dressed in white came and introduced themselves, and the man

said, "So, David, are you ready to roll on out of here?"
He was large, around six feet, two inches and around
three hundred pounds or more. He had a kind voice
and appeared to be a jolly fellow. I thought about how
happy I would be working instead of being in this use-
less state. I had a small envy of him that I prayed God
would give me relief from.

"You know all about rolling," the woman said with a
cackle in her voice. She was fairly thin with black curly
hair. She seemed to be a few years younger than the
man she was working with, but I believe they were both
under thirty. She was above me, behind my head, and
seemed to be working on my IVs.

The air felt cooler on my face as we entered the hallway.
I was bundled up with blankets, so I was still overall
well-regulated temperature wise. It was brighter in the
hallway as well. The light had been slightly subdued in
my room, and I preferred it to the harsh overhead lights
of the hallway. I could not tell too much of what was
going on around me as I was flat on my back looking
up. I got few side glances to see my movers and my
Dad close at hand. Dad stepped up and followed me
as I supposed he wanted to know where I was headed.
The two movers brought me down the hallway toward
the elevator, just laughing away.

"You got a license to drive this bed?" my Dad asked.

"His license is probably revoked," she said slyly.

"That's okay," he said, "I have been driving these beds a long time."

"That's because you're old,"

"I prefer experienced," he said in return.

The banter was entertaining. I always did like things a little on the light side. After all, being sick was a heavy concept, and the frivolity helped to set a mood and give me a short break from my serious self. With those jokes, we made it into the elevator, and my dad followed. The man then said something I couldn't hear, and it made the woman laugh uncontrollably. At this, I was a bit disappointed, and I worked real hard not to play the "they must be talking about me" card. Being sick can often make one more self-absorbed than usual, but I knew I could fight this. Besides, it was more likely that they could have been telling a more personal and perhaps an inside joke that was none of my business. It was overall a pretty smooth ride to the neurology floor. I was getting healthier. Coming out of intensive care, coming out of a real danger of dying, I was now entering a new stage of recovery.

When I first went up to neurology, I was in a bit of a panic. I had a pretty good-sized, white-walled room. There was a bed, my IV pole, a nightstand and one of those tables that fits over the bed, so the patient might have easy access. I still had no access as I had no movement in my arms.

"I can't stay here as the nurse's desk is so far from here, and I can't use a call light."

"It will be OK, David. We will check on you," said a tall, thin nurse with a pleasant smile. Inside, I was becoming overwhelmed with fear. I was filled with so many "what ifs" that I'm sure fear filled my face. I was almost hyperventilating, and I even felt a tear forming in the corner of my eye.

"I will see if I can move you closer for your own piece of mind."

With that the nurse left, and I was there with my parents who were now seated on the two comfortable-looking, bright blue chairs.

"Tomorrow's Friday. So I suppose that the powers that be will be out for the whole weekend, including Labor Day. Not much will get done in this stretch as I am sure they will pull the pin early tomorrow," Dad said.

I was thinking about being helpless in this bed and that something would go wrong. The truth be told, I was just built up with anxiety, and fear was building up in my guts and shoulders that I was just starting to get a little feeling in. I was overcome with a fear of abandonment. Looking back at it now, I probably didn't have to worry, but in that moment I really felt fear. I was having a tough time trusting. Sure, the nurses would have less time for me, but I would be cared for. My Mom and Dad would visit quite a bit, and they would make sure my needs were met. Joan certainly was my advocate, so I would be treated fairly. I still feared the night. I would be defenseless and unable to communicate. My limbs didn't work, and my voice was fairly weak, giving me no way to call out. The thought of God that brought me comfort. I wanted to focus on Jesus for he could bring me victory over my fear. I was double paralyzed. My body suffered from GBS, and my mind suffered from fear of the future.

I decided I needed to say a little prayer in order to calm my nerves. I closed my eyes and asked Jesus to be with me even more than I can imagine. I really needed to feel his presence washing over me. After a couple of minutes I opened my eyes and just looked at my parents sitting there calmly.

"Did you get a little nap?" said Mom.

"Sort of," I said back in a weak voice.

The nurse came back with good news: I would be moving closer to the desk. Relief started to wash over me, and I knew I would be able to trust that things would work out. It felt like a cloud was lifted, and my prayers were answered. I would soon be in a safer place.

Chapter 10

A Tale of Two Families

"And looking around at those seated in the circle he said, 'Here are my mother and my brothers, for whoever does the will of God is brother and sister and mother.'" Mark 3:34).

One thing I have done for the past twenty or so years was Fantasy Football. This was a hobby of drafting individual National Football League players from different teams. When you played games; your score was based on the individual scoring that player came up with in a particular week's game. As the owner of a Fantasy Football franchise, you are faced with injuries, poor performances, and sometimes the sweet taste of victory. Late August is prime time to draft your players. When I first started, I would draft from someone's home, and after that I played online for many years. I was never great at it, but I made it to a few Super Bowls, and I think I might have won one league.

I worried that with no arm movement, I wasn't going to be able to play this year. Since I had been in and out of consciousness the last few weeks, my brother-in-law Tim reminded me of the upcoming season. The hospital had Wi-Fi and Tim said he would bring his laptop, so with his help, I could draft a team even with my disability. He made the arrangements, and the day came to draft my team. He came in with Joan and Andrew.

"Hi, Uncle Dave, I hope you feel better" said my usually shy three-year-old nephew Andrew. He was the only child of my sister Joan and her husband Tim. Joan laid out some toys for Andrew to play with as Tim settled in to prep me for the draft, positioning the screen, so we could both see.

"Are you manly men all ready for your little draft? Joan asked.

Tim and I were laughing at some of the opposing picks and trying to apply strategy to a game randomly. This was fun doing something that seemed normal with people I enjoyed. Tim was totally engaged, and it was great to have Joan and Andrew in the background. This was the kind of family life that I looked forward to around the holidays. Joan and Tim are great people, and I'm proud that they are related to me. I really felt that way about all my siblings. They are an active group with all the members sharing a desire to live life to the fullest. With Mom and Dad as the leaders, I am blessed with a great family. I haven't always been able to spend as much time with them as I would like, but I cherish what I have. I'm not married to a woman, but to a whole Church. I have no biological children, but many call me Father. This prompts me to have a deep love and concern for those who make up my birth family.

We were drafting in the middle rounds when there was a knock at the door. I looked over at the door, and there stood Archbishop Nienstedt. He walked in with his black suit and a shiny chain visible across his chest, connected to the hidden pectoral cross of a bishop. The Archbishop is a tall, thin man with a substantial crop of white hair. He appeared imposing, and I felt helpless in my bed. I couldn't shake his hand or stand up straight like I thought I should be able to do. I greet him rather nervously, both surprised and intimidated that he was here.

"Father David, how are you feeling?" He seemed a bit awkward when he asked this as I sensed a bit of hesitation in his voice. I mused that he was as nervous to see me as I was him. I had always had some difficulty with authority, and the Archbishop had quite a reputation for being a bit standoffish.

He was empathetic and seemingly more human than his stern German personality usually showed. He listened with concern as I told him about the progress I had made and described where I hoped to be heading soon. I explained about the step-down hospital of Regency and the hope of ending up at Courage Center.

The Archbishop is my father in my vocation. Priesthood is far more than a job; it is a brotherhood. We say that we are always a priest in the order of Melchizedek, who was an Old Testament king and priest who stood as a precursor to Jesus Christ. This figure had some characteristics of the Christ, who came into the world. So all priests are my brothers, and along with my Archbishop, make up a family.

Now I hadn't always been faithful to this family. I struggled in seminary and my early priesthood, so I often felt less important than most of my contemporaries. I felt shame around them. I had good relationships with a few priests, but overall there was a real disconnect between most priests and me. A while back, I went through my CaringBridge site and realized there were a fair number of priests who communicated with my family and me through this form of social media. A few visited, and a few others wrote cards, but many didn't seem that affected by what had happened to me. I did find out once I recovered that many priests prayed for me and wished me well when it came to clergy events. So there was brotherly care, but I was normally pretty isolated from my brothers.

I vowed to work more on this. Due to the distance, I don't always take the time to be at as many events as before because they were mainly in St. Paul. I make other trips to the Twin Cities sometimes up to three a week that I didn't always feel like making another trip. I have prayed about it often, and I must report progress. In 2012, I was still far from feeling like an active participant in the brotherhood.

I didn't always agree with my Archbishop, but I did obey. He deserved respect, no matter what position he took. You don't have to like the guy to work for him. I gained a great deal of respect because he made an attempt to relate to me. The Archbishop spoke of Fr.

Joncus, who at one time had GBS. He mentioned that Fr. Joncus had an even rougher time than I was having. Knowing that the Archbishop wanted me to recover and wanted me back in ministry was comforting. I wasn't one who craved attention from the top brass, but his presence was kind of nice.

"Well, I can see you have family here, so I will leave you, and I will keep you in my prayers," he said.

When I was hospitalized, I saw a kinder, gentler Archbishop. I sensed he was sort of using my family as an excuse to duck out, but he is a busy man and he did come to visit. The Archbishop often makes me nervous, but for this short time I felt that he really cared.

Tim finished drafting my team and told me all about what I had missed. Joan and Andrew continued to play in my room after taking a few breaks. Tim packed up the computer, and the Hlas family headed out. They left me tired and thankful. I was happy to have a team from Tim and support from the man I pledged obedience to. My birth family and my priesthood family serve different needs I have as a whole person. I knew I wasn't going through this illness alone. GBS separated me from all the normal activities of my life, but families united me with humanity, so I could stay grounded and connected as I moved toward recovery.

Chapter 11

Chosen in Regency

"Put on then, as God's chosen ones, holy and beloved, heartfelt compassion, kindness, gentleness and patience." (Colossians 3:12).

It was the first week in September when I took up residency at the step-down hospital named Regency. I was now conscious most of the time. Various activities filled my days like working with staff, entertaining many visitors, or getting in some good prayer time.

At least part of the day, I spent watching television. I couldn't channel surf because my arms didn't work, so I watched the same channel for long stretches. One of the shows I watched a lot was *The Voice*. I saw hour after hour of preliminaries. The people would sing with the judges facing away from them. There were three judges. One was a soulful black man, joined by a white country singer with full twang, and the third was a woman pop singer. If one of the judges liked the voice, they could turn around and have a chance to put that performer on their team. It reminded me of people being picked in gym class, only this time it was singers. I was horrible at gym class so was often picked on the lower end. This didn't exactly build my ego. These performers would sing, and sometimes no one would turn around. At other times, all three would turn. Dreams were being dashed right before me. This was difficult for me to watch.

Sometimes I felt my hopes were dashed. I would get depressed about not being able to move. People around me would be encouraging, but sometimes I would still feel abandoned. I had this nagging fear that I might never walk again. I would ask God over and over why this was happening to me. I would never get a clear answer, but there would be nuggets of hope brought before me. It would be the smallest thing like a smile from one of the nurses or a kind word from the person taking out my trash. It was even the cheery visitor, some cousin or parishioner, who came a long way to see me. I would delight in these uplifting occurrences, and they were signs to me of God's everlasting mercy. I felt I would be chosen to move again; I just had to be patient.

Sometimes I was challenged when I ate; I was forty-eight years old and had to be fed like a baby. This was humbling, but I got sort of used to it. Nursing assistants were overworked and at times made horrible feeders, as they just wanted to get it done. The best was when I had a visitor around meal time. My brother, Rich, the engineer, had great pacing and skill to make the luscious forkfuls of goodness glide into my mouth. He was a pleasant feeder, and it brought back images in my mind of feeding him when he was very young.

I also longed to feel human again. I couldn't do any of my own grooming, and it bothered me. I'm used to shaving every day, leaving no facial hair. Once, I wore a mustache for a short time, but, hey, it was the eighties.

Now, with a month's growth, I really needed a shave. I couldn't handle a razor. That was something so simple, but I was dependent on someone for nearly everything. I was a bit embarrassed to ask a family member to shave me, so I asked a nurse's aide, and I'm glad I did.

The aide who gave me my sponge baths a number of times was a man named Ari. Ari was from Iran and in his late twenties. He had olive skin and jet black hair. When it came to the baths, Ari was fast but thorough, and I always felt clean when Ari helped me. One day after a bath I asked, "Ari, do you think I could get a shave?"

"You are looking a bit scruffy, but I think I can help you out," he said with a little laugh.

"That would be great as it's also a bit scratchy."

"And you can't itch, so I'll take good care of you and will shave you when I come back. I need to get to a few other patients first."

With that, he was gone. This man moved fast in whatever he did. I wondered if this was just the way he was or if the job required it. His mouth and hands were equally fast, and I had a reasonable thought that Ari was a type A personality. He was like a human tornado. I believe he rolled from room to room at breakneck speeds. True to his word he returned in about an hour.

Ari flew in the door with about three3 sample cans of shaving cream and about three of those disposable razors. Slightly out of breath, he placed the shaving equipment on my bedside table and said, "I'm back, and we're going to get down to business."

He applied a hot washcloth to my face. This felt so good, not too hot, and very soothing. Next he applied a very thick layer of shaving cream. It felt great as he worked it in to my bothersome facial hair. I asked him if I was keeping him from something, and he replied, "I am busy, yes, but I always have time for my friend Dave."

I asked Ari about school. In another conversation he had shared that he was taking business classes at a local junior college.

"It's fine. We started last week, and I am already tired. You know, you work full time, go to school full time, and where is there time for yourself?"

"Wow that sounds busy. It must be kind of hard."

"It is hard, but there are many more opportunities in America than there were in my home country. That was why, at sixteen, my brother and I got out."

"You must have been brave to enter an unknown land."

"You're brave for letting me shave you."

The whole time we were talking, he glided multiple blades over my face. He smiled and laughed while he made smooth work of my face. He finished by again placing a warm cloth over my face and then drying it with a fresh towel.

"Best work I could do with the equipment I have. You like?"

"Yes, I feel like a new man! Thanks a lot, Ari."

With that, he cleaned up and blew out just as quickly as he came in. I was selected to be cared for and despite feeling helpless, I felt the care. The whiskers represented the trauma I went through due to GBS. Even though I had been a pretty independent man, I was now dependent, and the whiskers would leave my face only with help.

About two weeks later, I was able to shave on my own. I was looking in the mirror at my face while seated in a wheelchair. I felt proud when I thought about where I had come from. My parents had bought me an electric razor. Gone were those cheap razors as I now let this marvelous machine glide over the contours of my face. As I shaved clean, it was now done more independently. This small matter was contributing to the bigger picture of what was happening in my life.

God was present during my time in Regency. I felt his presence in the calmness of my days. While Methodist was a blur of life-and-death activity, Regency was more filled with serenity and inactivity. There was quite a bit of alone time that brought forth much conversation with God. I longed to get better, but in listening to stories about my time at Methodist, I was grateful for how far I had already come. I felt chosen to go through this healing that I saw as a gift from God.

One day, early in the morning, my physical therapist and occupational therapist came together. The PT was in her late twenties and had shoulder-length, straw-colored hair with an air of quiet confidence. The OT was probably about my age with short brown hair and a pleasant smile. After some warm greetings, the three of us looked at my arms, and I slowly raised them up. I had never done this since the onset of my illness. I felt great jubilation and not really knowing what to say, I simply said, "Touchdown."

"Oh great job, Dave!" they said in unison. That was real movement. I couldn't wait for more exciting things to come. Unlike the unchosen in *The Voice*, I was now starting to be very chosen on my road to recovery.

Chapter 12

Souperman and My Life as a Priest

"In my God who gives me strength I have strength for everything" (Philippians 4:13).

My favorite nursing assistant, Arla, came bouncing into my room with the mail in her cheery disposition. She had an inviting smile with her tight curls, dark skin, and dark blue uniform. "Who are you, anyway? I swear, you get more cards than there even is. Oh sorry, I didn't mean to swear, Father"

We exchanged smiles. I was humbled as I realized one of the main reasons so many people write to me is because I'm a priest. God has given me so many blessings in my life, allowing me to connect with many people. It is rather mind-blowing. Besides the cards, there was a long tube, and I asked her to open it for me. Inside the tube were posters from school children. Arla held up many pictures of smiley-faced figures wearing priest clerical clothing. "We'll get these masterpieces up on the walls, Father."

My favorite was a picture of what appeared to be Superman with the title "Souper Dave." I like soup, and they serve it a lot in the hospital, so it only seemed fitting. Superman was my favorite superhero growing up. He is known for being strong, fast, and heroic. I love superheroes because of the action that surrounds them, and they often teach morals. I have occasionally used them as examples in preaching. During this illness, I tried to be Superman, and I knew I would triumph over GBS and grow as a person.

I could tell that Arla really liked this poster, too. "Oh for cute, gotta fly, Father," she said with a squeal and exited rapidly.

With so much time on my hands, I reflected on how Superman had also been an image of what I wanted my life to be. I thought of my childhood, remembering how hard it was for me to be super on the farm I grew up on. I was a farm kid who was never any good at farming. I remember being in junior high and having to face an irritated Dad. "Why are there so many marks on the garage, especially on the track the door uses?" he said.

Dad knew the answer as it had been me who had ruined the garage door and other parts of the farm. Usually I used the bucket of the loader tractor to do the damage that I let happen because of my poor eyesight and lack of attention.

"It's hard, Dad" I would say, nearly in tears.

"I know it is, but you have to be more careful. Concentrate on the job at hand." He would lecture me on this subject many times, but I never seemed to learn. I always thought he was mean, but I'm sure he was at a loss in what to do about his oldest son who was daydreaming much of the time.

I always longed to be super. In my mind, I was the great general, athlete, or cowboy. I had quite a few manual labor jobs. Most of them don't exist much anymore, like stacking small bales of hay or cleaning manure with a pitchfork and wheelbarrow. Now there are large bales and skid loaders. I worked hard, and I learned the value of hard work even though at the time it was pure torture.

"You don't need to drive the tractor today, Dave." Those words of my dad came as a relief. I would stand there in my tee shirt full of holes and my patched jeans scared I might wreck something. I had such a fear of machines and would be so tense when he wanted to teach me about them.

"Why don't you go out and bring the sows that are about to farrow to the farrowing house," he suggested this as an alternative project. These were the pregnant sows that were very close to having a litter. This was something I was good at. I liked working with pigs even though they were pretty stubborn at times. I felt more in control around the pigs than I did around machinery. Animals were far more exciting to work with. I have always had a great appreciation for animals.

One place I felt really comfortable was at church. I loved the mass; I almost never thought it was boring. I hung on the words of the priest and always seemed to get something out of the homilies. I would some-times lose focus, but I l enjoyed the bright colors of the clothing the priest wore and the bells that rang at the important time of the mass. The bread and wine were becoming Jesus, and I really rejoiced in this.

I was thrilled to become an altar server when I reached fourth grade. I dressed in my long black cassock that fit my body like a robe, and I wore a white blousy sur-plus over it.

"You boys look sharp all dressed up to have the best seats in the house," Fr. O'Connor mused as we got ready to process for mass. I was a bit nervous because this was my first time. "You will ring the bells at the right time, won't you, David?"

I nodded confidently. I felt good having him reassure me in an action that I would do often in my life as a server. I believe that anytime we perform a ministry at mass, we serve both God and his people.

I didn't date until college at the University of Wisconsin River Falls when I started to gain some self-confidence. At that time, I wasn't thinking much about the priest-hood. Then when I was a senior, I had a big breakup with a girlfriend of about two years. I started hanging out at the Neumann Center, which were the Catholic houses and chapel right next to the University. That spring I got to know Fr. Bob Olson who comforted me in my grief over the loss of my relationship.

One night after our men's intramural volleyball team, the "Holy Cows," lost yet again, we were drowning our sorrows in ice cream in the Neumann Center when Fr. Bob strolled in. He wore a baby blue sweater over his clerics, which are the black shirt and pants of a priest. He had a muscular build with jet-black hair and a constant smile. "I think there might be a couple of priests in this group," he said with enthusiasm.

The half dozen or so of us looked at each other and got real quiet after the good Father spoke. A quick thought flashed through my head: was he talking about me? No, he must be talking about someone else. Maybe it was Joe? With his blonde curly hair and killer smile, he seemed awfully popular with the ladies, but he had a quick wit that I bet would make him an excellent speaker. Tom might be one. He humbly got attention with his large frame, straight brown hair, and the ability to get along with everyone. He was also super smart and would be great at the studies in a seminary. Was there any chance Fr. Bob think I had what it took to be a priest? When I was praying in the chapel that next Sunday, the thought of priesthood came again, but I dismissed it. It lingered with me for four years until I finally applied to the seminary.

During the four years after the University, many wonderful experiences also happened to me as a Catholic young adult. I remember giving talks to spirit-filled teens who seemed to hang on my every word. I loved teaching confirmation and helped with two mission trips. I also liked the support I got from fellow volunteers that knew I was interested in the priesthood. Once

I announced that I was entering seminary with the hope of becoming a priest, I suddenly became more popular. I believe it was because people saw priesthood as a noble profession.

I had a food science degree, and after working a couple of years in Quality Control, I got a job as an assistant manager of a restaurant. I had been treading water in my management job, and now I seemed to be focused on a different dream. I learned a great deal in the food industry, but I never felt at home like I do in my vocation as a priest.

When I went to tell Fr. Bob that I had been accepted into the seminary, I asked him if he had remembered talking to our group of volleyball players one night four years ago. I even asked if he was talking about me. He said he did remember, and no, he wasn't talking about me. I just smiled and realized God had used Fr. Bob's words to plant the seeds of my vocation. The fact that I had carried around the secret for four years told me I had something in common with Superman who had kept his identity hidden from so many. In the seminary, I could be so bubbly on the outside, but I kept my true emotions hidden. I still kept some secrets, which are still being revealed—even to me.

Becoming a priest seemed almost magical. That first year was filled with many blessings. I felt so at home in the ministry. I was able to help others while letting Jesus be the center of my life. A priest tries to meet people where they are and let them know just how much God loves them. I believed I had the greatest job possible, being able to lead prayer. I also tried to help people realize just how relevant God was in their daily lives.

Superman had super powers he learned to use throughout his life. He had to train and learn how to use these special powers on earth. One power I developed was public speaking. I was never afraid of getting in front of people. I wasn't a natural at speaking, but I have always liked the challenge. I have worked on it my whole life.

Sports were popular in my growing-up years, so I wanted super powers in this area. My athletic skills were minimal, but my parents also let me try a variety of things. I failed a great deal in many areas. I was in three high school plays and never got the lead. I was in many speech contests but could never get above second place. I am not writing this for pity, but the lack of success shaped who I was. I don't have an entitled bone in my body, and I am always looking to improve.

I dreamed about being on the radio. My dream died when I flunked the entrance exam for Brown Institute. Much of priesthood has me talking for a living, so I don't feel so bad about not fulfilling my radio dream. I have better dreams like winning hearts for Christ and making people consider their faith more. Preaching has always been a top priority for me. I believe it is the most important action I take all week.

I remembered, in particular, one occasion I presided over a couple's wedding. They were beautiful people both inside and out. He in his black tuxedo and short black hair looked truly in love with his wife to be. She was breath-taking, wearing a conservative white dress, all beaded up. Her makeup was light, really drawing out her natural beauty, with high cheek bones and a sweet smile. Her hair was up, making her look even more elegant than she did when we met for their marriage instructions. They both seemed to really appreciate my spiritual advice. We laughed a lot and got into some extremely deep conversations where time seemed to stand still. Now they were standing together with their right hands joined, and they repeated after me as they declared their love for one another. I remember feeling like I was a part of something really great. I was doing my part to let them know that God was witnessing their love. I love weddings and really see them as a way to spread God's love and touch on evangelization.

Superman had a costume and a cape. As a priest I wore clerics. They have a little white tab on the front of the neck. This was from the days men wore a removable collar on their shirt. Priests wanting to turn their back on worldly pleasures wore the collar backward. I struggled at times as a priest. I haven't always turned my back on the world; in fact, there were times I turned away from God.

Was feeling alone a consequence of being a hero? Not really; in the case of my priesthood, it was an opportunity to draw closer to the source of all love. Jesus was my constant companion, and prayer is how I recharged. I was an introvert at heart as I gained strength from being alone, but I was never really alone. God has allowed me to be a part of people's lives at the most important times, and this was super. God was really in charge, but he used me as an instrument like a divine writer composing a satisfying sonnet. I had a role to represent the greatest gift to humanity. Alone, I was far from adequate, but with his presence, I was undefeatable.

When I was lying in my hospital bed at Regency and wondered if I would ever be able to be in ministry again. I thought about what I would do if I wasn't a priest. A writer, working in geriatrics, or possibly hospice. When contemplating these choices, priesthood was always the top choice. I missed the people and preaching the Word of God. When people visited, I was given glimpses of what I was missing. I believed that if I ever made it back to ministry, God would make me even more super. But I knew I didn't have to be super. I just had to be me.

Chapter 13

A Short Journey and a Beautiful Beginning

"All who call upon me I will answer. I will be with them in distress. I will deliver them and give them honor." (Psalm 91:15).

F rom the ambulance door of Regency hospital to the ambulance door of Courage Center was said to be one mile. Before the illness, it would have been an effortless stroll with a good friend on a beautiful sunny September day. I pondered this as I was lay in my bare hospital room as I awaited on my move. I was upset that we didn't take a short wheelchair ride with a small Metro Mobility bus instead of the high-priced ambulance ride. I confess that I grew bitterer over time, especially when I got the bill. I think the wheelchair would have been possible if the physical therapist had let me try one more time at the end. She made one lame attempt the week before, but none after that. I know I made progress. I suppose I should cut her a little slack in that she didn't see GBS very often, and she had no idea what a fighter I was.

I was upset, but I turned my anger into fuel and tried to recover even faster. Just like I embraced the cross of being paralyzed, I needed to try and not be discouraged when things didn't go as I would have liked. For the most part, I was good at this. Knowing what I know now, I could have proved that therapist wrong.

The ambulance attendants seemed professional as they entered my room in their white shirts with dark patches that told me there were from North Memorial. They were also dressed in black pants and black shoes. They took me from the confines of my hospital bed rather easily and brought me into the high-tech stretcher. I was ready for the hope and challenge of the Courage Center.

We moved through the mostly sterile white corridor in the hospital. The red and white ambulance took up most of the doorway out. The roll took only a few minutes, and I was well entertained. A few things made these ambulance workers humorous. One said, "Don't worry Father, we got ya; we have only dropped a few."

And the other said, "We better get you strapped in real good for the long trip."

One was tall and thin, serving as the driver. The other one was fairly short and a little portly. He rode with me in the back, hunching down by my side. When they picked me up from my room, they reminded me of the old comedy team of Stan Laurel and Oliver Hardy. I saw Laurel and Hardy reruns growing up and thought they were just hilarious. They were an odd couple of men who didn't say too much but were real funny with their slapstick actions. One time they had to move this piano up and down hills, making for some really funny scenes. I imagined being a piano and being taken by stretcher from Regency to Courage Center. That would have been more fun and perhaps a bit cheaper.

Once we were in the vehicle, the shorter "Hardy" attendant looked at me and said, "You are kind of a rare bird, having this Guillain Barré disease."

"That is what I am told—something like two in 100,000 a year."

"That sounds about right. Do you know how you got it?"

"No, the doctors never really said. I was worn down from traveling in the southern part of the United States."

"That might have done it."

"Some of the hotels I stayed in—let's just say they looked better on the Internet."

"I could see that one, I have stayed in some pretty bad places myself," he said with a smile, and we both laughed.

Thoughts of my road trip were very freeing. It was just me and my bright blue Ford Focus on the open road. That was in contrast to the small quarters of the back of the ambulance. The late September air was still fairly humid, and the sun shone brightly through the small windows of the emergency vehicle. This small cocoon will take me on this minuscule ride between two campuses that butt up to each other.

"Well, your maiden voyage is about complete." The "Laurel" character said from the front of the ambulance.

We stopped, and in a minute or two, the bright light shown through the open door of the ambulance. We appeared to be under some sort of car port. My personal comedy team got me down, so my wheels hit the sidewalk, and I could feel the nice warm air as I viewed the car port from my back.

"Easy does it, Dave," the Stan Laurel-like attendant said.

"We'll get you there, David," Oliver Hardy said as he grinned, "After all, this is door-to-door service."

As we rolled into the elevator, he asked, "Are you nervous, David?"

"Maybe a little, but I am ready to take the next, I mean, first step."

"Thatta boy; they will work you hard, but you seem up to it."

The elevator soon reached the first floor, and we rolled down a long hallway to see more bright light and people scurrying about. As I entered the threshold of room 115, I noticed two beds with a pulled-back divider and off-white walls with a TV hanging on each half of the room. They moved me all the way to the window side and gently transfered me to bed. We exchanged pleasantries, and the duo departed.

In seemingly no time, my mom joined me in my new room. My half seemed smaller than my Regency digs. Mom had a salad with her, and soon I had a little lunch. I was now starting to feed myself. Things were cut up for me, but I was able to take nourishment.

I got to wear real clothes there, and Mom brought me what I needed to enter this new stage. My body felt a little constrained in pants and shirt as opposed to the free-flowing hospital gowns I had grown accustomed to. St. Paul talks about a new man being clothed in Christ, and I now felt new.

Mom and I were engaging in conversation when all of a sudden, there was a knock at the door, and I heard my name. There was the shuffling of more than one person as they went through, passing my roommate's bed as they came into full view of my bed. I saw two attractive women in their late twenties. The taller one with light brown hair said, "Hi, you must be Dave. My name is Tina, and I am going to be your primary physical therapist."

I was thinking of myself as a lucky man as she came off both caring and confident with her athletic build and professional dress, wearing a light blue striped shirt with gray slacks. She had a great complexion with little or no makeup and had bright blue eyes and a constant grin on her face. I wouldn't have called her bubbly, but she had kind of a magnetic personality. "This is my helper, Kara, and we're going to get you in a wheelchair."

"You are, are you?" I was taken back by what she said because I had been flat on my back for over a month. I said this, being skeptical, but took it as a personal challenge. I knew getting into a wheelchair meant progress, but I was blown away that this woman was going to get me there within thirty seconds of meeting me. I believed she saw some doubt on my face, but the more I listened to her, the more I felt I could take on the world. My doubt turned into a smile, and I sensed Tina liked my attitude.

She looked at me long and hard and said, "I would like to ask you if you have any goals for your stay at Courage Center."

"I want to walk out of this place," I said more confidently than I really was.

"Wow, that's a great goal," Tina responded.

"I'm a Catholic priest, and I want to get back to ministry in my parish."

"You might not be able to get right back, but we'll help you make it. You are going to have to work, but you sound motivated. I am actually Lutheran, but I will help you anyway," she said with a smile. I think it is funny that she is a Lutheran. We never know who God will send.

Kara, who wore black slacks and a purple top and had a lovely rounded face and dark brown hair, disappeared out of my view and returned pushing this silver wheelchair with a light blue seat and matching back. It looks fairly used and may have seen its better days.

"Here is your chair, Dave. It might not look like much, but then again I predict you won't be in it long," Tina said.

Kara put the chair in place, and Tina made the bed sit me up. They quickly worked together to lightly lift me to my chair with the Hoyer lift. It was a bit of a struggle as I was basically dead weight. I wanted to help, but as the norm had been lately, I was helpless. They finally got me seated, and I was happy, but it felt a little weird to be out of bed. Tina made sure I was buckled in. I thought about how strange it was to be upright. I didn't really like it that much. I tried to give myself a push by pushing down on the wheels. I just rocked a little.

Tina smiled and said, "We'll have Kara push you for now, but soon you will be going all over the place on your own. I am confident you will heal fast. I have seen a few Guillain Barré patients, and they had done well. It just takes time."

We rolled out of the room and were greeted by nurses and nurse's aides in brightly colored scrubs, along with fellow patients in wheelchairs. I was thinking that this is friendly place to be, and I was glad because they told me I would be there around six to eight weeks. Tina walked alongside and probably was talking to me, but I was pretty zoned out as I took in my new surroundings.

Kara got my attention when she said, "Dave, did you know you have a roommate?"

"Yes, I'm told an eighteen-year-old Hmong boy."

"That's right. His name is Tou, and he should be back from the hospital tonight."

I thought about how incredibly young he was to be in a place like this. I wondered about his injury but thought better not to ask. Tou and I would share much over the next six weeks.

We reached the end of the hallway, and I now faced two elevators. Tina hit the button and almost immediately the right one opened up, and we rolled in. The elevator car was reasonably full with the three ladies and my chair, but the ride was brief. Tina explained, "The cafeteria, the PT rooms, and other residents' rooms are on ground level. We just left first floor that has your room, outpatient therapy rooms, and the doctor's offices. Here you will see Dr. Warhol your physician at least once a week. You may also see her physician's assistant some of the time. The first floor also has the main lobby and the pool you should be in, in a couple of weeks."

I grimaced at the thought of the pool. Water and I weren't exactly friends. I didn't say anything, hoping she would move on.

"Here we are at the Creekside therapy area. You will be here a lot," said Tina."

We first rolled into a small entryway that was for patients to meet their therapists in. There were a few chairs, but mostly small spaces that I bet wheelchairs went in. Straight ahead, the door was cracked open to reveal offices that I learned the therapists used. We rolled into a room to my left and saw two large raised mats, an apparatus with rails that I bet was for walking, and a ton of therapy equipment. There were balls of different sizes. There were several walkers, a bunch of different weights kind of cluttered the area. There were was a set of small steps. There were even a few things I had no idea what they were. I just took it all in, and Tina kept quiet, allowing me to look it all over.

"You will get a chance to use most of that equipment. This is the room where the majority of your therapy will happen," said Tina.

"This looks like it will be fun. How will I get to my appointments?"

"Kara here will bring you to and from appointments until you are more mobile. She will put you into the hallway, and I'll bring you into this room, so we can work hard."

"So, how often will I come here" I asked.

"You will have physical therapy six days a week. You will use this area and some surrounding areas for occupational therapy. Shari will be your main therapist, and you will meet her tomorrow."

I continued to soak the sights of my new home. I felt like a kid who started at a new school. There was a small amount of fear, but there was an even greater amount of hope that this would be a real place of growth.

Chapter 14

A Pair of Physical Therapy Firsts

"But seek first the kingdom of God and all his riotousness and these things will be given on to you." (Matthew 6:33).

Since Tina was on vacation, I saw Anna for the third time this week. With her help, I transferred easily from my chair to the raised mat in Creekside therapy room. She had on a purple shirt and jeans while sporting a button about wearing jeans for charity.

"You get to wear jeans," I said with a smile.

"You pay some money and get to wear jeans—a real bargain."

Anna was strong; she used very little effort to make the transfer. She is muscular with a pleasant face and short brown hair. She now put my head toward the wall while I was on my back and she used the position to begin stretching my legs.

"Dave, you are a little tight today."

"I tell you it is not from overuse. As you were saying yesterday, that must have been some wedding."

"So beautiful on the farm I grew up on. My family and I really transformed the farm into a great wedding site."

I cringed both from the pain and from the fact that my religious upbringing wasn't happy with outdoor weddings. I knew that bringing up the wedding would make her happy. Just then she started to push down on my leg. "OK, Dave, give me a little resistance." I try to push with all my might. She continued, "Push harder. There you go; that's it. You are getting so strong."

"Thanks, I don't feel all that strong."

"You are. What I like about you, Dave, is you bring the effort."

She has me push with the other leg. Just then my mom walked in with a big smile on her face. She was my biggest fan, wanting to be there for everything. "Your schedule said you'd be here. Is she working you hard?"

"I think she is about to," I said.

I was getting a bit of a workout by offering resistance. I wore out pretty quickly as that is part of the disease. It was a part of my illness that I tried to fight through. Anna stopped the stretching, and I sat up on the edge of the mat with my feet firmly on the ground. "You are going to stand today," Anna said and smiled.

I said a quick prayer for Jesus to be with me, and I also trusted in the pretty, young, professional who thought I could stand. She placed her hand on my shoulder to steady me, and I slowly called on my legs to support me. I was a bit like a newly born baby calf that was struggling to get my legs to work. I checked my balance, and boom, I was standing. I said a quick prayer of thanksgiving and said, "Look, Mom, no hands."

"O my gosh," my mom said as she rose from the chair she sat in.

"I knew you could do it," the confident Anna said.

"I have a hard time believing I did it," I said back in amazement.

"Tina is going to be proud," said Anna with a little enthusiasm.

In less than a week at the Courage Center, I was standing. I went from stretcher to wheelchair to standing since August 11, and it was early October. I was on my way to recovery.

After a few more days of therapy, I was back with an entourage that consisted of both my parents and my sister Joan. I looked forward to coming to therapy each day because I never knew just what great things would happen. I stood last week, but now I felt like the sky was the limit. My sister squeezed my shoulder with reassurance as we waited for Tina to appear.

Tina was dressed professionally with gray pants and a gray, white, and soft pink thin-striped blouse. She flashed a smile and said, "Good to see you, Dave. I see you brought your people."

"I sure did.'"

"Are you ready to get started? I've got plans for you."

"I am ready for anything."

"I know you are as you are one of my clients who actually likes therapy, and your enthusiasm is going to help you. Let's get you on the mat." She brought the wheelchair over to the edge of the raised therapy mat, and with a little effort, I hopped over to the mat. "Nice transfer," she said. Tina worked out my legs a bit. I felt the tightness in my muscles as she worked them over. "Do you still have that great amount of pain?"

"I do, but it is not too bad."

"OK, let's see if you can stand again."

I scooted to the edge of the mat. I start to really try to concentrate. I pictured myself as an athlete, trying to pull off a maneuver. I really wanted to perform this movement in front of my family. I knew I could do this. Now is the question of actually doing it. I went ahead and readied myself by trying to think through the move. I was going to let my legs do the work, but I was going to fight for total body control. This standing stuff was not for the faint of heart. Something I used to do without thinking was now a great challenge.

Tina grabbed my hands to steady me and I started to really balance myself. She was smiling the whole time as I seemingly supported myself with her lightly holding on. I was a bit skeptical, but I really stood again.

"It is all you; I am barely holding on."

I surveyed the room, seeing balls, mats, walkers, chairs, and all kinds of brightly colored stuff that I might use in the future. I focused on Tina as I was starting to gain confidence as she slowly let go, and I was there for a bit. Then I started to go down on my rear end. She grabbed on, so I didn't do a total plop, but I did come down pretty hard.

"That was a good one," she said with encouragement.

"Yeah, I thought it wasn't half bad."

"Ready to do it again?"

I got up again this time with even more confidence. With a spirit of competition in her voice, Tina said, "This standing stuff is starting to get pretty easy. I think you should take a step this time. Don't worry. I will be right here to help you. Let's start with the right."

My family watched with hushed attention as I told my brain to lift up my right leg. Tina had one hand on the cloth safety belt around my waist and one arm on my shoulder as she stood facing me. I made the move with my right leg, propelling myself forward. I wobbled a bit, but Tina was right there to help me balance.

"Nice one!" my mom said with enthusiasm.

"Good, Dave!" Joan matched Mom's intensity.

Dad was silent, but I looked up to see an approving smile on his face.

"All right, Dave; let's try the left" Tina said with authority. This leg was a bit harder to lift as those muscles were weaker than the right. I'm naturally right-handed, and that whole side had always been dominant. I was going to move forward with my left. I called on the muscles, and they responded as I took the next step.

"Now the right again," Tina said, urging me on. I picked up the leg and surged forward. She again caught me as I wobbled. I noticed my progress and was feeling ecstatic. "Kara, step over here, and let's get Dave down for a rest." Kara took the other side, and they backed me up those few steps, and I plopped down on the mat. "Nice plop. Your balance is pretty good. If you're up to it, I would like to keep going. Rest a bit, and then we are going to give those muscles another workout."

I was out of breath and tired. This took effort, and I knew the GBS wanted me to stop, but I knew in my heart that I would continue. A couple of steps was nice, but I wanted to walk. I let my body rest. I started to pump up my mind. This would be done if I put mind over matter as I went through this exercise.

"Let's do this." I said.

"Kara, you take the left side. We are going to take the weight off of you, Dave, so you can take a few steps over to the bars." Tina directed me toward the parallel bars that were about waist high and a few feet away. This is super exciting as I have pictured myself using them in my mind many times. Kara came over and placed a hand on my belt and my left arm. Tina did the same on my right side and said, "OK, right leg." I moved at Tina's command. I did this with more confidence as the women helped me with balance. "Left leg." I moved, and we took several more steps before we reached the end of the bars.

"OK, we are going to let go, and you will have to steady yourself on the bars." Tina said with confidence—more confidence than I felt as I looked down the twenty feet of bar.

"Here goes nothing," I said as the women released me, and after a slight balance check, I steadied myself on the bars.

Tina kept one hand on my waist as a safety net. "OK, Dave, let's take a few steps."

I moved along the bar kind of wobbly like a newborn fawn. I made progress as one foot went in front of the other. Totally braced on the bars, I made my way to the other end.

"Now here is the tricky part; we are going to turn you around," Tina said as I switched my hands on the bars and moved myself around with plenty of help from Tina. I did a major balance check and looked down the bars again. I moved with greater coordination and ease as I trudged down the bars. Each step was a strain. I felt winded, but I moved on against my desire to stop.

"Whoa, take a break, Dave. You are doing great. We will get you back to your chair. You did an awesome job. We will definitely build on this for next time. What do you have to say for yourself?"

"I feel real good."

Tina acknowledged my family and said, "He did a great job. Be sure to tell him that. This is a major milestone. He is making so much progress that it is hard to believe."

There were smiles around the room as I got back to my chair. Kara looked at my dad and said, "Do you want to take him back?"

"Sure, I can do that," he said with pride in his voice.

In that moment, I was filled with a healthy sense of pride in myself.

Chapter 15

Rock Star

"Magi from the east arrived in Jerusalem saying, "where is the new born king of the Jews. We saw his star rising" (Matthew 2:2).

Today was the day. I was a few weeks into my stay in Courage Center, and now I would be in a Care Conference to try and decide my future here. I felt comfortable in my wheelchair, but I had a way to go in my recovery. I was now standing on a regular basis and even stepping along with quite a bit of assistance. I thought back to the beginning and realized how far I had come. Only a short while ago, I was taken off the ventilator, and now I was going to be evaluated on what I had done here in this short stay. I was nervous about what my next steps would be. Would I end up in a nursing home or would I be able to stay here and get better? Would they let me go to parents' house? Would that be good for me, and could I handle the obstacles of the stairs to my bedroom? All these questions worried me, and some of the answers I had could come to a head at this conference.

I had a fairly free morning to pray. My life has always been a constant connection to God, but in the hospital, I would often do nothing and rest with the Lord. Jesus who loves me just as I am. I was given an incredible chance to just "be." So often we are caught up in doing things, and now I realize GBS gave me many opportunities to just "be." I would sometimes just sit and pray prayers of thanksgiving. At times, I even thanked Jesus for my failures, as they served to be great teachers. I realized that I had many more successes when I was patient with myself. God works slowly at times, and I just needed to let him work. Another part of my prayer life were my required daily prayers. With a little effort I could now handle my prayer book. This wasn't easy, but being back in the rhythm of the Liturgy of the Hours gave me stability. This was prayer five times a day. I was good at Morning Prayer and usually worked toward completing all the hours. This type of prayer was started by monks in a monastery, but now all priests and religious communities did some form of this prayer.

The conference was to take place at 11:30, and a little before 11:00, Mom and Dad came in. I was happy to see them. They were smiling and tried to be chipper. Dad was in his blue, short-sleeve shirt and khakis—a different attire than the faded work jeans he usually wore. His mop of brilliant white hair was missing the ball cap he had on most of the time. Mom, not letting her hair gray, had on a blue top with some white flowers detailing the shirt and blue slacks. I looked at them and wondered if this whole experience didn't age them some.

"I brought your laundry," Mom said as she immediately started putting it away. Aids did laundry for most of the rest of the folks, but I had a really dedicated mom who did my laundry, and I was extremely grateful for her work that greatly benefitted me.

Dad stood on the left side of my bed and said, "We'll have time for lunch right after, won't we? You get pretty good chow in this place." I really enjoyed it when he and Mom stayed to eat with me.

We conversed a while longer, and then about three minutes before the conference was supposed to start, Joan flew into the room. She looked a little stressed. She missed quite a bit of work because of me. She was at work more now that I was getting better, but you could still see the stress in her as she shouldered my cause.

"Are you ready for this?" she said with a smile in her voice.

"I'm a bit nervous for this conference," I said in a shaky voice.

"You shouldn't be because you're doing great. I just want to help you with the system here."

Part of my concern was, would I be ready to be on my own? Being a priest is demanding. Would I be able to overcome my physical barriers? I knew my heart had grown, and I knew I would have much to say in my preaching. I was a little nervous about being out of practice. Did GBS dull my mind? I didn't think so, but I still worried about it. Why did I waste time with worry and not simply trust? Was my faith that weak?

Marie, my nurse that day, poked her head into my side of the room, telling us the time for the conference had arrived. I was now in my wheelchair, and we moved to the room next to where the conference was held. Joan pushed me into this rather plain-looking room with white walls and ceilings. Several small paintings of landscapes were on the walls. Two mahogany tables ran parallel with the medical people behind one while we sat behind the other. There were several feet between us. The tables had white chairs and a space for my wheelchair. The social worker identified herself and welcomed us to the conference. She is a nondescript woman in her gray sweater and black pants. Dr. Bonnie Warhol was there as well, dressed to the nines complete with white lab coat. I like Dr. Bonnie as she was neat in appearance and witty in assessing things. She was a good doctor, always explaining things to me, and her presence put me at ease.

The social worker started the meeting with a smile as large as a jack-o-lantern. She droned on about the purpose of the conference and some other stuff. My own social worker sister, Joan, spoke for me. The conference felt surreal to be there and the talking sort of went over my head. The talk turned into medical mumbo jumbo, and I started to check out, so I was glad to have Joan there. When I heard Joan talk, I would sort of drift slowly back into the room. I wasn't always clear about what everyone said, but I could tell that Joan was holding her own.

I totally popped back in the conversation when the social worker, in her gruff voice, started to praise me.

"David, you have done so well here." She said, "David, are you with me?"

"Yes, sorry. I just get worn out."

"No problem; it's just part of your illness. As I was saying, he is making a great deal of progress."

"I have seen some real strength build up in the arms, and even the legs that came in really weak," Dr. Warhol said.

"The reports from the therapists look good," the social worker said.

I wondered what they wrote about me. They always seemed so positive. Was this really the case, or were they just trying to be nice to the old sick priest? I needed to have a better outlook. I really felt that God was helping me.

"Tina wrote many good things about you. In fact I really liked this. She called you her 'rock star,' as you were blowing all the goals she set for you out of the water. She was so impressed by your progress that she said that you would be out of here in no time," the social worker chimed in.

I smiled, soaking in the praise and feeling delightful. "Rock star" was a term used to identify greatness. Rock stars were famous, and they were achievers in the music world. Tina was saying that I was a "rock star" of rehabilitation.

Joan asked the social worker meant when she used the words "no time."

"We would like to keep David three to four more weeks if possible," Dr. Warhol said. "It all depends on insurance. The therapists will write up the care analysis in order to keep David at Courage." the social worker added. This was great news. I would have some time yet to recover, but I was slowly healing.

Despite difficulty, I now considered this a positive experience. I wanted to share how God has changed me as a priest and as a man. I now knew life-changing illness first hand, and the pastoral care I would give would never be the same. I was a very active and dedicated priest who wanted to be a rock star, like Peter was a rock for the early church.

"Rock star" was, for me, more than just a cute name. This nickname defined my way of life. As a priest, I am the "face of faith" to my people. I was a "rock star," not for my own fame, but for the person of Jesus Christ. I am on the front line, preaching the Word and offering the Sacrifice of the mass. St. Peter was the rock the Lord built his church on. I am one of the tiny rocks that keeps the church going, despite all the obstacles she has.

My triumph over GBS is one of the best things that ever happened to me. I knew that in this meeting, but I needed to experience the rest of my journey to turn it into a reality.

You might wonder why I chose to call my experience with GBS a triumph. I was eventually glad I was able to go through this experience. GBS was my cross to triumph over, but this cross was very small compared to the Cross of Christ.

We left the conference and went back to my room. Mom placed her hand on my shoulder, Dad showed a big smile, and Joan gave me a hug as I sat in the chair. Joan left to go back to work. Watching her walk away, I thought about when I would be walking and when this chair would be totally unnecessary. I was making progress, but I wanted to be back to normal—whatever normal was.

This would end up being my last conference, but Joan continued to advocate for me until the end. Tina's "rock star," comment made me smile. From now on, everywhere I went in the facility, the comment would follow me around because it was in my chart. It was fun to hear it, and I thanked Tina for the strong report. Tina, the athletic-looking former college basketball player, simply looked at me and said, "You deserve it, Rock Star."

Chapter 16

Tou, My Roommate

"Friends or neighbors are timely guides" (Sirach 40:20).

I rounded the corner to my room and tasted the food with the smells. The cooking was Asian, and it tempted me, being fried and spicy. When I entered my roommate's side of the room to get to my section of the room, I saw Tou and his family feasting. There were seven of them crammed like sardines into the A side of the room. Besides Tou, his four brothers ranged in age from a small toddler all the way up to a teenager; all had short-cropped, jet-black hair of similar style. The brothers' tan skin and brightly colored clothes made them visually enjoyable. The group was busy wolfing down the tempting delights. I figured the older man and woman were Tou's parents. His dad was well muscled and strong, like a man who had done much physical labor. He wore a bright green shirt and jeans. His face had pock marks and wrinkles near his eyes. I thought we must have been about the same age, but he could have been younger as labor can age you. He appeared wise with his gray temples.

Tou's mother looked powerful in her compact frame and the way she carried herself. She was definitely in charge of all those boys. She had a matronly look about her with long dark hair, brown eyes, and an inviting smile. "You want some food?" She said in slightly broken English.

I looked into her caring eyes and nodded, even though I had just come from lunch. "Wow, this food looks wonderful."

"You try egg rolls. I have fresh and fried."

"I'll take one of each please."

"You probably not want hot sauce; it may be too hot for you." She said this with a chuckle. I had a hunch she was right. I was a true Minnesotan who sometimes thinks ketchup is a little spicy. OK, that is an exaggeration, but I was pretty sure her sauce was too hot for me. She placed the fresh-looking rolls on a paper plate and handed me a plastic fork. "You want some fried rice?"

"You bet! Did you make this all yourself?"

She answered with a grunt that sounded a little like "ya" and flashed me a big smile. Then she quickly turned and said something firm in what sounded like her native tongue. I thanked her, and she shot me another smile as she turned back to her children.

I retreated to my side of the room with my precious morsels in my lap and maneuvered my wheelchair the rest of the way through his crowded side of the room. Once on my side, I gobbled up the food because the tastes were out of this world. The cold roll was like a salad with the thin paper-like wrapping. The fried egg roll and the rice were better than anything I ever had in an Asian restaurant. I was now super full and felt a little sleepy. I gently transferred onto my bed.

I was glad the curtain was three quarters of the way closed, giving Tou's family a little bit of privacy. I could hear the active dialogue but was clueless to the content of their conversations. The mom and I spoke a different language, the language of food. This language crosses many cultures. This was her way to show love. The gesture seemed like her gift for my caring toward her son.

A rustling noise on the floor by the curtain caught my attention. It was Tou's youngest brother. He was shy, but he smiled at me a lot. He was now laying on the floor directly under the curtain. He would look to his left and make eye contact with me and observe what I was doing. The little boy would then look to his right and see his mom speaking to her eldest son. Her long bursts of words were followed by a short quieter sounds from Tou. The youngest son would look back and forth at the different sides of the room. He would make himself dizzy, and this would cause him to smile and look straight up. He would then be in a world all his own. I was inspired by him because he tried to figure out our different worlds. It was east and west right in room 115. I was learning so much at Courage Center from learning to walk and dress to even getting a look at a different culture.

I remembered my first evening in my new room in the B section near the window with a beautiful view of trees and a walking path. The dividing curtain was pulled nearly wide open, so that I could see people who entered. My side was the fairly sterile room except my colorful Indian flags, a gift from my friend's adopted daughter from India. Hung also was a Minnesota Gopher gold towel from Dad, who recently went to a game. He knew how much I loved this hometown football team. I had just taken my 8 p.m. pills, when two paramedics came in with what looked to be an Asian boy. Nurse Nancy had told me to expect him as he was coming back to Courage Center.

As the ambulance attendants finished putting him in his bed, Nurse Nancy said, "Hey, Tou, welcome back! I would like you to meet your new roommate, Dave. He has Guillain Barré syndrome and is paralyzed a bit like you. He'll be trying to get better. We want you to try, too."

He looked a little frail, with jet black hair and big brown eyes. As the nurse left the room he said, "Hey, Dave, what you got, Gee something?"

"Guillain Barré syndrome. It attacks the nerves, causing temporary paralysis."

"That mean you get better, man?" I answered positively, and I wondered how much better he would get. I could tell he wanted to talk, and he continued. "That's cool. I had a bad diving accident. I was at a party showing off, and I didn't know how shallow it was when I dove off the dock. I hurt my back and neck real bad. I can't move too much."

"Wow, that is too bad. Can you feel your arms and legs?"

"Not down below my waist. I've good feeling in my upper body, but not great movement. I'm working on that. I'm getting better at my chair. I get a new one next week."

"That's cool. My chair is pretty junky, but Tina says I won't be in it long."

"O man, you have Tina, too. She's very pretty."

"Yes, she is." It was scary how much I thought about that.

"She's very funny, too."

"Yes, I really like her personality."

We talked for a while longer. He was a sincere and inspiring young man with an outgoing personality that was pretty much the opposite of me. He was Hmong and eighteen, and I was white and forty-eight. My heart ached for him as I realized he would have a tough journey ahead of him. We signed off after a while and he said, "Say, Dave, I'm glad you're my roommate."

Eventually Tou and I built a relationship through a photography class we took together. I remember the first night. About nine or ten students gathered in the TV lounge. The lounge was homey enough with a blue carpet and a few brown tables around the fairly large room. There were puzzles and games on shelves fastened to the walls and a TV with a combination VCR and DVD player hooked in an entertainment center that had seen better days. There were many VHS tapes of comedies and dramas from all sorts of eras. Many of them I had seen. I made mental notes about trying to watch a few in the future. Tom, the wheelchair-bound activity director, was there. He thanked us for coming. He introduced Angie, the cute twenty-something volunteer with short, curly hair and long legs. He also introduced Marsha, the instructor of the class. Marsha was in her forties with medium length brown hair and a large number of earrings. She was dressed in loose-fitting pink and blue pastels giving her what I would call an artsy-fartsy look. I would find out she was quite the accomplished photographer.

As Marsha spoke, as I observed rest of the room, on my right I saw Tou was just transfixed on her. He was laughing deeply at all of her jokes and gave the impression that he thoroughly enjoyed himself. On my left I saw that she was not connecting with many of the students. There was even quiet words of dissension among some of them. This was during a PowerPoint presentation of the history of photography. Before it even started, there was a long delay with technical difficulties. Marsha, Tom, and even Angie worked feverishly on the laptop and projector that were to be our visual aid. A couple of students left before the first slide even made it up there. Marsha's presentation was pretty dry, and she wasn't super confident. Several more residents excused themselves with thinly veiled excuses like needing to get medication or to get to bed. I heard from a woman who left because she was bored. I admitted

I thought it was a poor presentation, but I wanted to take pictures.

After the mass exodus, that left the smiling Tou, two fairly able-bodied guys from outside the center, and me. I later learned the guys were former residents who suffered from brain injuries. If fact, one them would take up residence again before I left Courage Center. Our reward for enduring the first part of the session was that Marsha and Angie brought out cameras. The two outpatient guys and I were able to use a regular camera, as our upper bodies were fully functional. On Tou's chair, Marsha mounted a bracket that allowed him to view the back of the camera, so he could see to take pictures. There was a switch connected to a gray tube that connected the camera. He could squeeze it to take pictures. It was a pretty neat set up, and it delighted Tou. I enjoyed taking pictures, but it was more fun watching Tou as he took pictures. He was way into this art form, and I felt like a proud parent seeing my son find some-thing he really liked. He slyly talked Angie into helping him. She focused her full attention on him, and he was loving it.

After Marsha saw that the other two students were set, she came over and helped me. She was very knowl-edgeable and was much easier to understand one on one than she was with the PowerPoint. We posed chess pieces and other shots around the recreation lounge. Marsha was giddy about photography. This was a look into her world.

The following week, the class met again. For this class, we were outside on the walking paths that I could see out the window of my room. There was quite a bit of room out there, and the four of us were all lining up shots.

"Taking pictures is fun, Dave," Tou said as he used his modified camera. He grabbed a nice shot of some trees and water on the center's grounds.

"This is fun. I'm glad we stuck with it," I said. There was a stream with a few ducks and a walking bridge.

"Dave, look over here. This is going to be the best shot ever." He was like a kid in a candy store, and I loved his enthusiasm. The early evening air had a slightly cool tinge to it. We were fighting darkness while the sun was going down behind the trees. I snapped a picture of the side view of the bridge that crossed the creek.

We went in the center and edited some of our shots. We would have an exhibit of our two favorite photos the next week, so in this session we finished getting them ready. I was so happy that my sister came to the show. Little did she know that I planned to give her my best photo as a Christmas present. The class was a welcome break from therapy.

The drawback to being Tou's roommate was that he needed so much medical attention. I often found it hard to concentrate on things, and it was even harder to settle down to sleep when there was so much going on behind the drawn curtain. At times, I think the staff thought the curtain was real thick and believed I couldn't hear their voices.

"Tou, we just bandaged you up and now you've made another mess," came the voice of an aide.

"I sorry. I didn't mean to," he said.

"That's okay. Look at this sore, it looks tender. Do you feel that?"

"I feel nothing down there," he said with a giggle.

"Oh Tou, let's get you cleaned up."

There was a small break of silence. I wanted to call out for assistance as I was in pain, but the aide was for Tou and not for me. We had the same nurse, and I wanted her to give me my night pills. They were for pain and sleep. I was just on the edge of really needing them. Finally the nurse poked through the curtain. "You alright, Dave?"

"I'm having some pain, but I'm hanging in there."

"What time do you get your meds?"

"8 o'clock, usually."

"Well, it is 9:20 now. I will run get those for you. I bet that pain is getting pretty strong. It has been a while since your last dose." She would soon be back with my drugs as I then would try and get some sleep.

I had to admit that I was a little envious of all the attention Tou got. When I would pray and realized just how lucky I was to be reasonably healthy. I asked God for forgiveness for my envy and lack of patience toward Tou and the staff. I wanted to get home and have my own room, but sharing a room built character and let me experience life in a way that my normal days as a priest didn't allow. I'd been told you never quite knew who was going to be your roommate. This time I learned patience and joy from my roommate, Tou.

Chapter 17

Nurse Know-It-All

"That God may afflict you and test you, but also make you prosperous in the end." (Deuteronomy 8:16)

"You must do something about those feet," the nurse said, after bursting into my room. She was a spitfire with sandy blonde hair and glasses that made her look like a school teacher.

"OK," I said a bit put off. I had just taken off my shoes and socks after a long day of therapy.

"They're in such bad shape. I see someone made a crude attempt to help this big toe, but it looks just awful. They should have taken the nail all the way out, as it's going to become ingrown again."

"A podiatrist worked on it when I was at Regency."

"Well, he did a horrible job. Another thing, you are going to have to keep those nails trimmed or you are going to have loads of foot problems. Look at how rough and chapped they are. Nothing short of a miracle will make them presentable again." She paused. At that moment, I felt responsible and full of shame. Later I realized that my response came from my own stuff, probably linked to some painful events in my childhood. I perceived her as a real bully, and this unfortunate event cemented my extreme dislike of her.

"Lucky for you, I have experience with feet," she continued. "I'm going to make them as good as new. I'll clip your nails and put lotion on your feet. I'll make a note in your chart for the other nurses you see at bedtime to apply liberal amounts of lotion on your feet. I'll help you, and you'll be better for it."

She did as she said, and my feet responded with marvelous results. The process of clipping and applying lotion was painful because of the neuropathy in my feet, almost like she was trying to inflict pain. But you couldn't argue with the results. The lotion was applied to my feet daily, and I even kept it up on my own after returning home. My feet were like those of a child.

That same nurse, Ann, was in charge of me one evening. She stormed into my room and said, "How can you stand it?" She said this in a loud voice, as she viewed my partially clothed body. I've never had a real healthy body image, but her curt remark didn't make me feel very good about myself.

"Must I discover every little thing that is wrong with you?" She said this about a pesky rash I had. I didn't reply because I was so physically tired; I just bit my tongue afraid of what I really wanted to say to her. My initial reaction was to scream at her, but I knew that would be the wrong approach. I felt the heat in my cheeks as I let her push my buttons.

Nurse Ann made me appreciate all the other nurses who cared for me during my stay. I didn't have much against her initially, but her overly critical and superior attitude drove me nuts. I nicknamed her "Nurse Know-It-All," a title I never used to her face or to anyone else at Courage Center. I did use the name with a few friends who never met her; it was a way to blow off steam and get some sympathy. She would talk down to me for my health problems and then meticulously tell me what was wrong. I couldn't stay mad at her for long because she was good at what she did. I would try to pray for her, but there would sometimes be tiny tears because I couldn't let go of the disdain I had for her.

Her unkind and brusque approach toward me was confusing. Her loud voice used to ring throughout out the corridors, telling jokes. She was warm and friendly to almost everyone else. I could hear her caring approach to Tou on the other side of the closed curtain. She would joke around with him with a real sense of the familiar.

Once Tou said to her, "Good to see you; you are so funny."

"O Tou, you are too kind. I like coming to see you. The nurses and I will make the skin on those bottom sores as good as new. We'll carefully put on the salve on your precious bottom."

"Silly, you not have to be careful; I don't feel down there."

"I always want to be careful with you, Tou, as we hope you might end up feeling there someday."

"Tell me again about nursing school, and all those tricks you played."

"Perhaps another time, my friend. I need to see my other patients."

When I heard her leave and shut the door, I said to Tou. "You think she's funny?"

"She's very funny, always making jokes." I thought about that for a bit. "Nurse Know-It-All" was also "Nurse Jekyll and Hyde." Tou continued, "One time when you were gone, she had me put red jello in my mouth and had me call for Nurse Amanda. When she saw me, I let the jello run out of my mouth. Amanda looked at me in shock. Then Ann jumped out from behind the curtain from your side. Amanda screamed loud. Such a funny trick!"

"I bet it was funny for Amanda."

"Ya, ya." My sarcasm was obviously lost on him. "She is so great. I wish all the nurses were like Ann."

I couldn't share Tou's enthusiasm. I pondered why she treated me different than Tou. Was it my age? Was it the fact that I was a priest? Sometimes people treated me unkindly because of my profession. That may have been because of bad experiences with a priest or an anti-Catholic bias that exists in Lutheran Minnesota.

From that moment on, I started to pray for Ann, asking that she be blessed. I also started to compliment her more for all she was doing for me. I told her she was a quality nurse because her nursing care really healed me. When she treated a small rash, she was gentle and downright cordial. I thought she was totally out of character from what I had experienced her in the past. Near the end, she really started to grow on me. When I was ready to leave Courage Center, she gave me a big hug, and was I ever surprised.

Tou showed me the goodness of Ann. Prior to having GBS, I would have written Ann off. She would have continued to be "Nurse Know-It-All," and I would have continued to think poorly of her. Tou served as an agent of God, who taught me to remember to love those who persecute me. I blamed Ann for the way she treated me, and it looks like it may have been a defect in me that it made it easier for her to be cold. I was made teachable by an eighteen-year-old Hmong boy, and I was a better man for it.

Chapter 18

The Italian Dinner

"Amen, amen I say to you will weep and mourn while the world rejoices" (John 16:20).

The men's club at Sacred Heart Catholic Church has always put on an Italian dinner as a fundraiser. My sister's husband, Tim, had to work at the event as he had in previous years. Joan invited me to the dinner, and of course my three-year-old nephew, Andrew, was with us as well. I was very excited not having to eat Saturday night supper at Courage Center. The meal was usually a replay of the blandest and least popular of the food we had been served that week. Instead, I mounted my walker and headed for the car transfer into Joan's SUV.

We arrived at the Sacred Heart, but we had to park quite a distance away. When healthy, I wouldn't even have noticed it, but with a walker, the distance felt like a mile. We bought our tickets, and the wondrous smells of the Italian spices and warm garlic bread led us to the serving area. It was your basic church hall with white walls, accented with brick to give it an ordinary, slightly institutional look. There were red-and-white checkered tablecloths on numerous tables. Men in white shirts moved rhythmically around the room, serving up salads and hot plates.

122

We asked for a table for three and a friendly man with a big belly looked for a place to seat us. We saw Tim, busy at the task of serving. We wanted him for our waiter as Andrew wanted to see his Daddy, but Tim's section was full. Joan and I sat across from each other, and Andrew sat in a chair that was high at the head of the table.

"You like my church, Uncle Dave?" Andrew asked. "You feel OK, Uncle Dave? You hungry, Uncle Dave?" The boy peppered me with questions like cracked pepper on a salad.

I smiled and said, "Thank you, Andrew. I'm ready to eat and feeling good in your nice church."

"Andrew likes Uncle Dave," Joan said as the boy smiled in recognition. "You make his prayers every night. We pray for Uncle Dave, right, Andrew?"

"Yes, Mommy," he said with a giggle in his voice.

A tall man slapped down salads that looked fresh topped with Italian dressing. Then a man in his 50s with a mustache came and asked, "Would you like wine with the meal?"

Joan nodded, and I was a little hesitant, but then I smiled and Joan ordered red wine, which ended being a nice house Merlot.

"By the glass or by the bottle? If you want more than one drink, the bottle is a better deal," our waiter said.

"Bottle." Joan shoots me a look, and I smile back.

I'm not much of a drinker, but, hey, who doesn't like wine with pasta? When we were almost finished with our salads, a waiter arrived at our table. "Hot plates!" He presented us with a heaping plate with noodles, red sauce, and cheese, along with two meatballs and two chunks of steaming sausage.

"And for you, little one," he says as he serves a smaller plate to Andrew.

The food looked and smelled fantastic with a hint of oregano. The red sauce had a tangy flavor, and the noodles were only a little past al dente, but I loved them just the same. The meatballs were tasty, though not as good as Mom's. The sausage were out of this world. It had the right amount of bite and blended well with the whole meal. This was a lovely change-of-pace meal that was absolutely full of flavor. The wine and conversation among the sounds of people talking loud and the faint sound of Italian music was great.

Soon our table had a familiar visitor. "How's the food?" Tim asked.

We nodded and tried not to answer with our mouths full. Tim also patted his son on the back in affection as he quickly went back to work.

With full bellies, we made our way back to the car and Joan drove us back to their home.

"Did you have a good time?" she asked.

"Yes, with visions of sausages still dancing in my head"

"I loved the meal, and it was relaxing to drink wine. It was a good deal for a good cause."

"I know how you like your wine," I joked, and we laughed.

The tingling and pain in my feet, which is pretty much constant, started to spike a bit. Joan started to get Andrew ready for bed and asked me if I wanted to write on my CaringBridge, the computer site where friends and family can follow the progress of a loved one. This seem like a great idea, so she gave me the password, and I worked my way over to her computer. I had a fast-rushing pain, and I typed through the pain. I was pleased with my entry. I thought it showed an update of my progress and included a big thank you for prayers. When I finished the piece, I sat there with my eyes shut as waves of pain flowed over me.

"You all right, buddy?" I heard Joan say, and I opened my eyes to see a concerned look on her face.

"I'm hurting, and I'm thinking the wine might not have mixed well with my pain med."

"That could be true. I'm so sorry that you're hurting."

"I want to go back and see if they can do anything. I just want to lie down for a while."

"Tim just made it home. He can be with Andrew. I'll take you back."

"Sorry, Joanie, I don't think I made a very good guest."

"That's okay. Get some rest and hopefully some relief from that pain."

My feet felt like a fiery mess of molten lava as I sat at my sister's table. I used the walker to make my way out of Joan's house. With the shooting pain in my feet, I gingerly made it into her SUV. It was just a short drive from her home in Crystal to Courage Center in Golden Valley. A fiery pulse burned through my feet. Joan and I were quiet during our trip. I kept reviewing my choice to have wine. It went great going down, but was it worth it? This would be a resounding no, if I believed the wine responsible for this horror. Later, I read my nerve pain medications have an alcohol warning. I tried to surrender the pain, but failed miserably.

Joan helped me into Courage Center, and I checked back in at the front desk of the unit.

"How was the dinner?" One of the bubbly aides chimed in as I signed the book.

"The food was great, but now my feet are in pain," I said.

Joan could see I was really hurting, so she said, "I think he's going to need more pain meds."

"We'll make sure his nurse comes right away."

I made it back to my room with the walker, and Joan helped me get ready for bed. After she left, I just lay in my bed engulfed in a sea of pain beginning in my feet and radiating throughout my whole body. I was glad to be lying down as movement added to the spiking of the pain. I also appreciated the dim lighting coming only from a small lamp on my nightstand that created a peaceful glow in a place that pain continued to pulse.

I'm not great at waiting when I'm in pain. That evening there were many patients on the floor and only two nurses. They had a big job. When I was just lying there unable to read and really not wanting the extra light and noise a television would bring, Tou had his TV on. Lying there in pain, I thought the noise of his TV was excruciating. So I'm sure what was only a few minutes felt more like an eternity for someone to come and help.

"Dave, are you okay?" I heard the voice of a nurse.

"I need some medication," I said with a little more force than I would have liked.

"I'll take care of you, Dave. On a scale of one to ten, where is your pain?"

"Eight, nine, I don't know."

"Oh dear, I can help you. It says here you haven't had Percocet since 2 p.m. and it's almost 9."

In that moment, I realized that this was no ordinary nurse. This was Amanda, one of my favorites.

"You hang in there, Dave. I'll get the pills."

"Thanks, Amanda."

"You're so very welcome. I'm glad to be your nurse."
Even in the dim light I could see the flash of her caring
smile. Amanda was a glimmer of sunshine in the dark
hole of my pain. Her smile made me smile, and in the
back of my mind I just knew things would be okay. The
wait time seemed briefer, but I was more than ready for
this drug to tackle my pain. I gobbled up the pills followed by a water chaser Amanda brought with her. She
lifted my thermal mug and said, "I'm glad I brought
water because you are bone dry. I will get you some
more water as you need to keep hydrated. The water
will help with the pain."

"Thanks, Amanda."

"Not a problem. You just drift off to sleep."

I didn't fall right to sleep. I tried to pray. I thanked God
for Amanda, Joan, and Andrew along with all those
who had shown me kindness. I think because I knew
relief was coming, I felt like I was starting to stabilize. I
tried to surrender the pain to the wood of the cross. That
was the last thing I remembered as I slept in the deep.

Chapter 19

Bad Day at Courage

"For he will rescue you from the snare of the fowler" (Psalm 91:3).

I heard a knock on the bathroom door. "Hey Dave, it's Rachel. Are you in there?" Rachel was the physical therapist's weekend helper.

"Yes . . ." I said hesitantly as I wondered why she was at my bathroom door.

"Dave, Brian wants to switch your 2 o'clock appointment to 9." Brian was the weekend physical therapist.

"What time is it now?"

"It's about 8:40, so you have twenty minutes."

I had just gotten up on this lazy Saturday morning. The staff let you sleep on the weekends. I resented my aides a bit for not coming into my dimly lit room sooner. I didn't get the service I once had now that I could do a little more for myself.

"I'm not sure if I can make it that fast."

"He said if you were a few minutes late, that would be okay."

"I'll try to get there as quickly as I can."

"Thanks a lot, Dave. We'll see you down there."

I could have complained, but she was as cute as a bug's ear with her curly reddish hair and her light complexion. She was very thin and tiny with a great smile. I didn't want to bother her as she had no authority to change Brian's mind. Rachel was a really good person. Later, I found out that Rachel had spent time with an order of nuns just to check it out. She saw herself more in line with the life as a physical therapist, but who knows what God has in store for her.

Rachel was kind, and Brian was smart to use her to deliver this appointment change. It would have been easier to say "no" to him, but I really wanted the therapy, and I would do almost anything to get to have this session. A great deal would have to happen for me to make it on time. Hopefully, I wouldn't have to wait too long for pills. I called them in ten minutes, before I went to the bathroom. I had also asked for some breakfast, feeling some hunger pangs. I wondered how fast they would get to my room. I would probably end up going by the coffee machine for a quick cup of "joe." If late, my "privilege" was less therapy time. To miss therapy time was not an option, if I wanted to continue to be a "rock star." Now I needed to get washed and changed before pills and breakfast. I had less than twenty minutes, and my anxiety started to shoot through the roof like Old Faithful at Yellowstone.

Brian wasn't my favorite person. He was pushy and full of himself. I only had him on Saturdays, and I remember being overjoyed the one day he was absent. I wanted help with walking normally. Neither Brian nor anyone else was going to get in the way of this goal.

Less than twenty minutes later, I made it down at the physical therapy room. Brian, looking vain as ever, greeted me. He had a big head of brown curly hair, with a muscular frame, and was dressed in dark blue workout gear.

"Well, well, right on time. Thanks for making the switch."

"No problem." This was a little lie, but I didn't want to let him think he rattled me.

"We're going outside, and you're walking with a cane."

"Tina never makes me walk with a cane anymore."

"I'm not Tina, and we're going outside to see how you do on uneven ground."

"Maybe I should just walk it without a cane."

"That you can do with Tina. Let's get going with the cane."

"Whatever."

"I don't like your bad attitude."

Right then and over those passing weeks, I thought of many witty comebacks, but I stayed quiet because he wasn't worth it.

For some reason, I walked with the cane with great difficulty. I think it might be that I'm so uncoordinated that I don't have the right rhythm with the cane. Tina tried me with a cane a few times, but we both concluded that it wasn't worth it. I actually did better trying to walk on my own. I was a newbie at walking. At first I often had legs like Bambi, but Tina said it was only a matter of time until I mastered it. She said, "You're going to walk right out the front door." For the most part, I believed her. There are certainly days I struggled, and this was starting to look like one of them.

Brian and I went outside through the automatic doors of the visitors' entrance. The air was cool and felt nice on my face. It was perfect weather for football. The leaves were just starting to turn, and there was a bit of moisture in the air.

"Do you want a jacket?" he asked. I noticed that he wasn't wearing one.

"No, I'll be fine."

"Are you sure? It's a little cold out."

"I'll be okay." I said, partly out of bravado, but I also realized I would be using precious time to go back and get a jacket. My room was quite far, and I don't move at blazing speeds with my walker. I knew he had more appointments on the way, so this would once again be on my time. If Brian had been thinking, he could have sent Rachel with the suggestion. Perhaps that was asking him to think too far ahead. Sometimes I think the reason I don't like him is not so much because of a meanness, but because of his dull wit.

Outside, I took a few gentle steps on the sidewalk just outside the door, I felt like I started out okay, but there was a little frost on the trail. This made the trail slightly slick, and I didn't know how I would do on the wooden walking bridge ahead.

Brian was the last person I wanted to have for company on this morning. Silence became my demeanor, but he talked endlessly, "Get your feet straight. You don't want to be walking with your toes pointed out," or "Get more rhythm with your cane. It doesn't have to be so hard and awkward," or occasionally, "That's pretty much it. Good job." He said these different comments while I walked, using the first two comments far more than then the third.

I did try, but I didn't make much progress. In fact, I nearly fell a few times. Did he think all of his talking was going to give me greater coordination? I was really missing Tina. She was much easier to work with. If I was struggling like I was now, she would probably make a joke. Then she might offer a different technique or something. She wouldn't have kept on with the same mantra: "Keep that right foot straight. Strike the cane with your opposite foot. No, that's not right. Let's try it again." He did this repeatedly until about my third time, I almost fell. We headed inside, and he sarcastically said, "I don't want to fill out the paperwork if you fall."

The outdoors zapped me of my strength, and I was mad at myself for my mistakes. Brian didn't help much, but I knew this poor performance was my fault.

Once back inside, we walked with the cane some more. I was more stable, and it got to the point where he wasn't being quite as pushy. Finally he said, "Is there anything else you would like to do in our session?"

"Sure, I would like to climb the stairs."

"You can handle those?"

"I can and just to make you happy, I'll use the cane, too."

"Atta boy, let's see what you can do."

I made my way to the bottom of the steps and centered myself on the first step as I also prepared my mind. I could do this. I placed one foot in front of the other and climbed the steps. I relied much more on the railing than on the cane. If Brian noticed, he didn't say anything.

"Keep it up; you aren't doing too badly," he called from behind me.

"Thanks," I managed, slightly out of breath. I summited the top of the flight of steps.

On my way back down the stairs, Brian stood there seemly all too proud of himself. I knew I was progressing, and I didn't need his approval. I still didn't like Brian, and I couldn't wait for the session to end.

Chapter 20

Spiritual Battles

"And if the bugle gives an indistinct sound, who will be ready for battle" (1 Corinthians 14:8)?

After my morning appointment with Brian, I sulked off to my room and pulled my room divider as tightly shut as I could get it. I just wanted to be alone. I lay down on my bed to ponder. All through my life, I liked to use my bed as a place of meditation. I got comfortable, and God spoke to me. Sometimes it was vivid videos in my mind, or it might be a strong feeling in my gut. The speaking to and listening to God had always been a big part of my ministry as a priest. I found homily ideas that way. I charted a course for the pastoral council or approached tough issues of pastoral care.

Psalm 63 states "On my bed I remember you. On you I muse throughout the night." I have done a great deal of pondering and musing most of my life. Now I needed to wrestle with my thoughts. Good versus evil right happened on my bed at Courage Center.

In these battles, I was under attack. Evil would tempt me, and I would have to surrender all the pain to Jesus so that he fought the battle with me. The existence of both good and evil seemed real to me. I recognized that evil wanted me to give up. The Devil wanted me to stop trying and go through the therapy halfheartedly rather than giving it my all. This didn't make any logical sense, but this was exactly how I believed the Devil wanted me to feel. He appealed to my weakness of not wanting to put in the hard work. He tried to emphasize the things I couldn't do. He wanted to frustrate me. Had I given in to the temptation; I would have felt relieved in the short term and lost in the long run. The Devil used every dirty trick in the book to end my progress. He appealed to me by using pain, hardship, and even people to send me down the wrong path.

I won't go as far to say Brian was the Devil, but some of the things Brian did brought out the worst in me. The smugness of his huge ego really got to me. He was probably a good and worthwhile human being. I was sure that if Brian and I had met in another context, we might have slapped each other on the back in friendship. Well, that was perhaps a little far-fetched.

I wondered if Brian represented that part of me that wanted to condemn myself. This made it harder for me to become whole again. In my past, I had trouble with authority, especially when it came from a man. The Devil knew this, so Brian was like every man I had resented.

I just prayed that the Devil didn't get the best of me. Lying on my bed I felt self-pity and hopelessness. Prayer was one tool I have to fight the Devil from desolation. I knew with the power of God, I could defeat the Devil. The Devil and I sparred most of my life. I hold my own, but he sometimes he caused setbacks and pain. Then I got a defeatist attitude. If I really wanted to win, I just stopped and asked God for help, and the Devil would flee.

When I was in college, I went through a Christian rock phase, and one of my favorite bands was Stryker. They had a great song that was called "To Hell with the Devil." I didn't swear often, but when Stryker screamed out the song, I sang along loudly with them when I was in private. In my room in the Courage Center, I needed a little Stryker.

As I battled the forces of evil, I tried to think about things from my past that were pleasant. Sometimes they were few and far between in my mind, but I wanted to be positive and run the race as if to win. Victory wouldn't be mine, but it was all for the glory of Jesus.

I had plenty of good allies in this war. I thought of my loving family who was with me every step of the way. Close priest friends came to mind because some of them I knew so well that I realized we went through some of the same battles. I cherished the thoughts of all the people I had served who took time to remember me. There were strong images that comforted me and gave me hope.

There were blessings shown by my three-year-old nephew. If I ever wanted to see hope; I pictured the unconditional love in Andrew's actions. He shared, hugged, and kissed better than anyone. That little guy was both dependent on us and, more importantly, dependent on God. He was a role model. Small children hold nothing back. When they are mad, they cry or throw fits. When they are sad, they cry and mope, but if we love them, they often show an abundance of unconditional love through smiles, kisses, and hugs.

I saw this very much also in the children I ministered to. They so energized me that I was overcome with a great desire to share my faith with them. They were so receptive and appreciative that in my heart I believed they understood the Paschal mystery far better than some adults. The evidence was in their bright eyes and smiles. Children still really give me a lift.

Liturgy was another area I found totally uplifting. Many times I pulled off a lively mass with my dashing deacon, attentive servers, an articulate reader, and inspiring music. We all worked together to praise God. I wanted to be pleasing to God. I would try and act in the person of Jesus, like I was ordained to do. I offered him in Word and Sacrament. This wasn't done just for me, but for the whole world. I wanted to engage the people present, who were a worshiping community. In the Eucharist, I offered Jesus Christ, Body and Blood, soul and divinity, to all who believe. The Eucharist has changed me into a better man, a man Jesus Christ meant me to be. The Eucharist is the ultimate weapon against the Devil. My leadership participated with others in the sacred liturgies of the Church. This helped me believe in myself and in my God who loves me. My heart ached in the absence of this. My illness separated me from the Eucharist.

Gratitude was also very important. I tried to be grateful for all God has given, which is far more than I deserved. I also tried to be thankful when things weren't turning out as I had wanted. This was trickier to do. God also came to me in unanswered prayers. Disappointments build character and shaped me into who I am. Sometimes this was very unpleasant, but often some growth came from suffering.

For example, during much of my healing I had nearly unbearable pain. I didn't ask for this, but I knew it was my cross. I was confident that God would not give me more than I could handle. My pain was minor suffering that I chose to link to the cross. We call this redemptive suffering. I offered this pain for the other patients at Courage Center. I offered this pain for the protection of the unborn. I offered it for all who are in need of God's abundant mercy, including myself. I linked my pain to the pain of Jesus. It was all for gain.

This experience of the illness deepened my prayer. It makes me grateful for all the other people who have prayed for me. Many expressed these prayers through my CaringBridge site. This was a way my supporters could be right with me. We were linked by prayer. This connection really helped my recovery. When I went back and read some of those entries from the early days, I was so touched.

I remembered getting a card from a couple that I had blessed on their sixtieth wedding anniversary. I believed that I was a conduit that God showered this couple with abundant blessings. Now their sweet little pink card with little flowers blessed me abundantly. The Devil fled at the mention of all those blessings

This late Saturday morning I sparred with the Devil well. I made another decision to keep fighting. I wasn't going to let anyone or anything get in the way of my healing. I was going to work hard at each and every therapy session, so I could reach my recovery goals. I still had battle scars, and I even knew that doubt would probably seep in again, but I was ready. I rolled over and saw that it was noon and time to eat lunch. The food would be enjoyable, but the fellowship with the people I shared meals with would be even more enjoyable.

Chapter 21

Erin and the Pool

"Are you unaware that those who were baptized into Christ Jesus were baptized into his death" (Romans 6:3)?

T hrilled to answer God's call, I was drawn into service of the Church. I was twenty-eight, and I had been accepted by the Archdiocese of St. Paul and Minneapolis to study for the priesthood. My formation that fall was to be at St. Paul Seminary in St. Paul, Minnesota.

I'm an alumnus of the University of Wisconsin at River Falls. On this warm August day, I was invited to a party with people I knew from the Newman Center, an organization for Catholic students, across the street from campus. After meeting at the Neumann Center, we car-pooled to a lake near Hudson, Wisconsin.

Since it was nearly twenty-five years ago, who was there is a blur, but I remember Marlene, a hearty woman from Chicago and her friend, whose name I believe was Ann. There were about a dozen people ranging in age from about twenty-one to their early thirties. They were fun people filled with laughter. When we got to the lake, most of the group ran into the water and cooled off.

I remembered walking slowly to the water and starting to wade in more gingerly than anyone in our party. I walked over to a group that was talking in the water that was about chest high. There were about a half dozen gathered here. We talked about the past, fondly remembering our college days. We laughed about Fr. Bob, the longtime chaplain of the Newman Center. He had a quick Irish wit he said he inherited from his mother. We remembered his words of wisdom and the "golly gee" that would come out when he didn't understand us. He gave inspiring homilies about his time in Northern Sweden. Fr. Bob had told the group my big news about the seminary, and this brought a lot of chatter.

"Wow, I think It's great you're going for the seminary," Marlene said with a smile.

"I'm so excited," I said with a healthy pride.

"I think you would make a great priest," Paul, one of the young men said. I wondered what he based that on. The thought quickly passed, and I enjoyed the compliment.

All of a sudden, man named Greg, standing near me started to convulse. He was standing higher on a rock, and as he was coming down, he was flailing his hands all around trying to keep his balance. One hand ended up my head, pushing me under water. I took in a mouthful of lake water and was gasping for air while I couldn't touch the bottom. The flashing thought in my head was "Is this it?" I thought this was the end of my life. The faces of my family were being pictured in my mind. I thought priesthood wouldn't be realized. I was confused, and these moments seemed like a lifetime.

"Dave, you'll be alright." Marlene's voice sounded like an angel, "Dave, Ann and I are with you. Jimmy's taking care of Greg, and we're going to get you to shore." She placed her hand on my arm. I started calming down as Marlene and Ann guided me to the shore. I was relieved to see Jimmy helping Greg who also appeared calmer. I learned that Greg had epilepsy and had a seizure probably brought on by the warm sun reflecting on the water. I was profoundly grateful for the women who guided me to shore. Exhausted, I rested in the sand.

When we made it back to the Neumann Center, we told Fr. Bob of the near fatal mishap that fortunately had a happy ending. Rushing toward me, Fr. Bob said, "Oh Dave, I'm so happy you are okay." He gave me a hug. I had been fairly close to Fr. Bob during college, and now we had a different bond.

As we got in line for hotdogs, Jimmy said, "I bet this hotdog of yours is going to taste really good. You must have a real zest for life now."

Zest was the farthest thing from my mind. I was happy to be alive. My vocational journey continued with my dream of priesthood. My fear of water increased by leaps and bounds. After that, I only went in a pool a few times.

Years later, at the Courage Center, when Tina told me I was going to have pool therapy, that afternoon at the lake flashed in my mind. I didn't say anything to her or to anyone else, but it felt like a lead balloon in my stomach. Tina told me I was going to work with Erin, who was petite and in good shape. She was a new mom whose baby was just a few months old. I once saw Erin after one of my PT sessions. She had a motherly glow, as a group of women fawned over her and her baby. Erin's red hair and pasty white skin and a great smile put me at ease like the Irish girl next door.

On the day we began, Erin pushed my wheelchair to the water's edge of this large pool. Looking out onto this vast expanse of water, I felt afraid, and my fingers began to tap my chair. She strapped weights on my ankles to help stabilize me once I got into the pool. Erin helped me stand while I kept my balance with my hand on the railing that lead me into the pool.

"Just walk with me, Dave" she said reassuringly. She took my hand and brought me into the water that was as warm as a newly drawn bath. I moved with caution on my wobbly legs, trying to let go of my fear and live in the moment. The water had a faint scent of chorine. The morning sun shone upon us through the large windows, and it felt warm across my shoulders. Using the handrail to support myself, I moved one foot in front of the other. I was now walking into waist-high water.

"Are you doing OK?" Erin said as I panted, shaking with fear, and I decided to rest from this short walk.

"Yes, I think I will be okay." I wasn't being truthful.

"We're going to gently walk from one side to the other" she said warmly. This was in response to the choppy way I had walked so far.

I got up on legs that felt like those of a baby learning to walk for the first time. Erin faced me and took my hands as she walked backward as I trudged forward. Each step was a struggle, but we completed the first length of the shallow end of the pool. Clients and therapist pairs were all around us. I started to plod back with Erin walking backward. Her movements were graceful, but firm, and I felt very safe in her presence.

"With a name like Erin, you wouldn't happen to be Irish and Catholic?" I said.

"Wrong on both counts. I'm Scottish and Lutheran, but many mistake me for Irish." I weakly smiled and shrugged, thinking we had less in common.

"You certainly have an Irish name."

"Say, Tina tells me you're a priest, and I think that's wonderful. I really like my pastor as he's a great guy."

"I love being a priest. It sounds like your faith is important to you."

"It is, and we make it to church quite a bit."

We turned and I wobbled, but her hand on my shoulder gently guided me back into place. I was nervous and clumsy, but I was loping along.

"This seems like a dance I'm not very good at."

"No problem, I used to be a dance instructor. I've got you covered; besides, you're doing great."

Erin and I chatted away during this first session until it was time to get out of the pool, and she maneuvered me back into my wheelchair.

On another session, a few weeks later, we ventured out into the deep end of the pool. There was a floating blue-and-white line separating the well-used shallow end with the ominous-appearing deep end. Even though I was in the water, I was sweating bullets. As we headed out, my body was as stiff as a board.

"You'll be okay, Dave. Just stick with me." I had an iron grip on Erin's hand. That gal wasn't going anywhere without me. I also gripped my flotation noodle, a bright red thin plastic tube-shaped device that surrounded me. I trembled and said a Hail Mary to myself and asked God to help me trust.

Then a moment of clarity came to me. As I started to trust, I was able to lessen my grip on Erin and sit on the noodle to gently float. Years of anxiety started to literally float away. I had found peace, and in that moment, I trusted God, Erin, and myself. I'm not sure if I'm completely confident with water, but God brought me through my fear.

Chapter 22

Occupational Therapy

"Take my yoke upon you and learn from me for I am meek and humble of heart." (Matthew 11:29).

My head occupational therapist was a short, fit, and attractive young woman with a dark complexion. Her name was Shari, and she was extremely good at her job. She quickly learned that my fine motor skills, such as handwriting, typing, and playing the piano were weak. Guillain Barré affected my balance and stamina.

OT time was a fun time because we often played games. We played Uno, and Shari pushed me to move faster and faster. A few weeks later, we played Jenga, a game with forty small wooden blocks. At each turn, you take out a block and stack on top of the tower, with three blocks per layer with the layers being perpendicular to each other. I had played it before my illness, but usually I was sitting down. Shari made me do it standing up. We also baked cookies. She made me do that standing, too. I knew Shari was trying to push my limits, and I liked that.

One morning, I faced a new challenge with another occupational therapist in the third session of trying to dress myself. I was in my room, trying to pull up my pants, and it wasn't working. My arms were weak, and my legs weren't much help. Aside from the pants thing, I was making good progress.

These sessions were done with Katrina, a fresh-faced late twenties occupational therapist. Katrina was strong but carried herself in a gentle and caring way.

I needed to get my pants on. Without help, I was able to get my feet inside them, but then I got tangled up. They were lightweight golf pants, which should have been easier to put on than normal pants. I worked hard. Could I do this without help? Why would something that I used to take for granted be so difficult? I was on the edge of my bed, sitting on my bottom with the pants about halfway up. I was trying to lift myself to pull them all the way up. Next to me, my roommate Tou's television blared CNN.

"Just wiggle a little. This will help you pull easier," Katrina said with a slight giggle.

"It's hard to move my legs," I complained.

"I know it is, but you can do this."

This was my second time trying to pull my pants up with Katerina. I had already tried three times with my aide, Jasmine. I failed each time. These women had to help me, or I would have gone the day with my pants half way down. I was going to get it this time. I was going get out of here being able to dress myself. I paused, took a deep breath, closed my eyes, and said a silent prayer. "Here we go!" I put a vice-like grip on each side of my pants. I then lifted up my bottom slightly, wiggled, and pulled the pants up.

"You did it!" Katrina said with enthusiasm.

I blushed and felt a wave of relief. I was filled with joy over this seemingly simple thing that I could now do. I also felt tired. Who knew putting on pants could be so much work.

About a week later, Shari had a new challenge for me. She led me to a backroom of the gym with the view of the garden. We stopped before a large blue board covered with small red lights, all off. The board was about six feet tall and five feet wide. The lights were evenly distributed on the board. I was to stand before the board, and as lights went on, I was to press it, and it would go off. It seemed pretty easy, and I wobbled some, but for the most part I did it with ease.

"That was good, but you can go faster. The board will go as fast as you want to go."

I pressed fifteen lights on that first try. That was pretty poor. It took twenty-five to show I had the reflexes to drive a car. I wondered if I would drive again. Life would change dramatically if I couldn't drive. I would miss out on rural living since I couldn't expect to be driven everywhere.

"I can do it!" I said as I braced myself for the timer to begin again. I tried with all my might. This time I attacked the board with more intensity. I really tried to push myself.

"Twenty-two," she said.

I readied myself again prayed that I could hit twenty-five. I really wanted to drive "Twenty-three. That's close; we can come back another time."

Later that same week, Shari said, "You want another shot at that light board?"

"I sure do!"

I was a little nervous as we drew closer to the board. I was focused now. It was 10 a.m., and I felt strong. I had a nice breakfast and prayer time, and I was ready to perform. When we stood before the light board, Shari gave me a firm look and said, "Okay, I'm only let you do this a few times. If you get more than twenty-five, we'll stop. I want to have you do a few more things before you are done with OT."

In the area of the board, I pushed aside "Walker Texas Ranger," my nickname for the dreaded walker and brought my body into a ready position squarely in front of my nemesis filled with lights. My eyes scanned the board, trying to imagine myself going fast. I was ready, and I turned my head to smile and nod to Shari. She smiled back and said, "You look ready! On your mark, get set, and go!"

The first light was up high and to the left. My left arm flew up, and I nailed it. Then there were two in a row to my lower right. The lights flashed everywhere. I flew over the board until I finally heard a buzzer, letting me know my time was over.

"Oh my, twenty-seven. Way to go!" I wondered if I now had a shot at driving.

Occupational therapy was part of my spiritual journey. While the primary goal of physical therapy was to get me up and walking, occupational therapy dealt with how I would live life. I had to be able to care for myself if I was going to be able to continue caring for others. I believe God gave me a mission to live out my life as a priest. I faced many trials in trying to complete this mission. GBS was a tough one as it is the only one that brought me face to face with death. My collective difficulties caused me to be tried by fire in order to be stronger. Occupational therapy gave me the strength and balance to help me endure any kind of hardship that might lie ahead.

When I was at my lowest point, I wondered if I would ever be able to function again. I was told I most likely would, but my faith was so weak that at first I was full of doubt. The earliest occupation therapy worked with hand movement that used equipment to strengthen my grip. With a good grip, I would be able to give my parishioners a firm handshake after a weekend mass. Going from being fed, to eventually being able to maneuver silverware in order to feed myself was a big accomplishment. I didn't want to stop there. I wanted to offer the sacred meal of the mass to the people who supported me with their prayers. I longed for us to once again be a community of believers, making memorial of this food of everlasting life.

Alterations could have been made for me to celebrate mass even with limited use of my body, but I longed to try and glorify God with all my strength. Just as I stood to play Jenga or to bake cookies. I wanted to stand as a beacon of hope behind the altar. Being able to bend down and pull up my pants was essential. I also trained to be able to go down on my right knee and genuflect in order to give praise with my body. Occupational therapy helped to make me whole again. For me, this was a necessary step toward realizing my own holiness.

Chapter 23

Tom and the Movies

"And when Jesus saw that he answered with understanding, he said to him, 'you are not far from the kingdom of God'" (Mark 12:34).

I concentrated on the small brown tile that whizzed by as I moved the wheels of my chair. I was getting pretty strong in my upper body, and I could lug the dead weight of my legs in my wheelchair that was my personal mode of transportation. As I exited the door, I felt the high afternoon sun warm my skin. Then a slightly cool September breeze prevented the sun from causing me to overheat. I wheeled my chair over to the vehicle that would get Tou, Larry, and me to the movies.

Tom, the activities director, was there to see us off. I felt reassured by his presence being slightly nervous about my first time out. Tom was also in a wheelchair, and his slick looking chair was a Cadillac compared to the model T I was trucking around in. His narrow wheels attached to a light frame showed the chair's superior engineering. Tom was probably in his late thirties, and he had an attractive confidence as he directed all of the activities. I was grateful to him as he had helped me obtain an absentee ballet so I could vote in all the local elections of 2012. This is but one example of how

Tom was a servant when it came to being a director. He literally knew what I was going through when it came to dealing with disabilities. His neatly cropped brown hair and strong-looking upper body gave him real "street cred" when it came to teaching me how to handle myself in a wheelchair. He made sure we could find our ride, and he told us he would meet us at the movies. He said he was going to drive his own car over there. I never asked Tom what he drove, but I pictured it being a classy sports car as Tom was a sporty kind of guy. He was college educated and friendly, giving him the ability to be good with people.

A small white Metro Mobility bus, with a lift, had room for three wheelchairs. Tou and I were first-time riders, so we hung back, and Larry, the aggressive veteran, lined his chair up to enter the lift first. There was a slight hum as Larry was secured to the lift and brought into the van. Tou went next with his nervous laugh. He said something to the driver, but I couldn't make it out. I just patiently sat in my chair and waited for my turn.

Finally the lift came down empty after the drive reappeared after securing Tou. He motioned me forward. "Put the chair right here," said the mid-fifties white guy with a few days' growth of beard. He was dressed in an ill-fitting blue and white uniform with a Metro Mobility patch. His facial expression and his oaf-like mannerisms showed that he probably had had a long day.

I pulled the chair in and with a jerking motion he brought me up and effortlessly rolled me into my spot. The muscular driver then strapped me down tight like I was getting ready for an amusement ride at Disneyworld. I thought about talking, but he was so efficient that I'm sure he didn't want to talk. I felt like a piece of meat with his rough handling of my chair. He treated me well, but so impersonal that I felt less than human in my chair. I resented this guy because he could walk, and I had to be moved around. I tried to dismiss the feeling as they were deep down self-pity, and I knew if I stayed in this frame of mind, it would lead me to self-defeating thoughts. I had been down this road before with my mood disorder. Self-defeating thoughts never got me anywhere but depressed.

The chairs were far enough apart that we couldn't really talk. I looked out the window at the cars and scenery I had been deprived of for the last eight weeks. I fantasized a bit about driving when I saw this red Mustang convertible pull up next to us. The balding gray-haired man behind the wheel looked like he didn't have a care in the world, and I longed to be like him.

Tom was waiting for us when we arrived, seeming curious about how the ride was. I didn't really answer the question as I wasn't sure how I felt at the time. I wasn't used to public transportation. I was used to being my own driver, in control of my movements.

There was a women in a power chair there with her young adult son with a barbwire tattoo on his upper bicep. We were technically with them, but Larry, Tou, and I hung with Tom who had been to this place many times before. It took effort for me to go from the sidewalk into the carpeted area. The floors at Courage were all pretty even and easy to maneuver. I struggled a bit here due to the sudden inclines and declines.

We made it to the box office, and when it was my turn to approach, I felt like a five year old looking up to the ticket taker.

"What movie would you like to see hon?" The heavy-set woman with gray hair and dark-rimmed glasses said in a friendly, but perhaps condescending tone.

"Argo," I said from my low position.

"$6.50 please." She said with a sappy smile on her face. I pulled out my money, and in that moment, I was over-come with the smell of buttered popcorn and the cool-ness of the conditioned air on my skin.

"He's with us," Tom called out, "so give him the VIP pass for free." I wasn't sure if this was a perk for guys in wheelchairs or if it was because Tom came to the movies so often. The VIP passes got us into this little eating area complete with a bar and sports-filled tele-visions. We were given a high price menu with $12 hamburgers, for example. I followed Tom's lead and ordered a meat and cheese appetizer. It was more than enough food with crackers and Greek olives complete with pits.

When it came time to see the film, we went into des-ignated areas for the chairs behind the first section of seating. Once inside, Larry and Tou started pulling out chips, granola bars, fruit, and candy bars from within their chairs. No wonder they only bought soda in the lounge area; they had brought enough food to feed a small army.

The film started, and I tried to get lost in the moment but was interrupted some by the munching of my fellow patients. Argo was a great film set during the Iran hostage crisis. This brought me back to my high school years when it was actually happening. I remember being on the edge of my seat, watching the hostage crisis in my parent's living room. I was now on the edge of a seat I couldn't rise out of. I was a hostage in my own chair.

The darkness of the movie theater added to a feeling of excitement. The darkness separated me from my fellow patients, and I was on the end of the row with two seats between me and the nearest wheelchair. The isolation was built up by hearing the other patients speak in low tones. No one was talking to me, and I couldn't even hear them clearly if I wanted to join in.

I let my isolation go and concentrated on the plot of the movie. Some of the US embassy workers, at the time of the takeover of the embassy by the Iranian militants, had escaped to the Canadian embassy and were hiding out there. The story is of a CIA agent back in the United States trying to get the group out of Iran as a film crew for a fake movie. He travels to Iran and tries to carry out the ruse with the backing of some real Hollywood producers. The movie was both funny and suspenseful as the plot continued to twist. It was a good story because even though you knew the group was going to make it out of Iran, the tension was still there to keep you guessing how they would do it. I wasn't surprised in the least when later on, Argo won the Academy Award for best picture.

I thought about like the characters in Argo. I, too, was on a quest. I was trying to escape from GBS. I had much help in this escape. It was a thrilling journey that kept me in suspense every day. Argo ended well for the main characters, and I hoped my little drama would have a triumphant ending as well.

Upon the conclusion of the film, I was tired, and my pain was starting to throb like someone was taking a hammer to my feet. I needed pain meds and would have to take some when I returned. I was hoping they would work if I was going to have any chance at sleep. It took me a little bit to gain enough momentum to roll out of my spot in the back row of the lower level. As I rolled out, I noticed the slopes of the floor. I was pretty sure that if I were walking I would have barely noticed it, but now I wheeled through and took notice of even the smallest slopes. There was one spot in the hallway by the elevator that was quite a climb. I noticed it on the way in, but it was easy to go downhill by regulating my wheels. I found it much more difficult to move up the hallway. It was taxing on my arms as I made the climb. Tom stuck by me, reassuring me I would make my way out of the theater.

We had to wait a while, and I pulled out into the early evening air. Larry and Tou smoked as we waited. Smoking is a disgusting habit, but I wasn't going to take the moral high ground with two fellow wheelchair

guys. I knew Tou pretty well as my roommate, but I had
only briefly met Larry. They never offered me a smoke
because perhaps they knew I didn't smoke. I also had
a hunch that cigarettes were taxing on limited incomes.
Larry had yellow stains on his hand to show that he had
been smoking for quite some time. Tou seemed like
a beginner, and his injury made smoking seem hard.
Was smoking a pleasure they could enjoy even when
other pleasures of the world seemed hard to grasp? I
knew I was getting out of the wheelchair soon. What
was their outlook? It didn't look good, and I'm sure
this was a desperate place to be in. One thing I envied
about smokers was their comradery. They seemed to be
a part of a club. I felt this way around church people
with coffee. I missed coffee with parishioners.

I was lost in my thoughts when Larry said, "Dave, how
did you like the flick?"

"I really liked it."

"I liked some of the action, but it wasn't very realistic."

"But it really happened. I remember hearing about the
story but not knowing all the details. The Iran hostage
crisis was a big deal at that time."

"You are like way old."

"I was in high school."

"Man, I wasn't even born yet," Tou said.

"So it was a bit nostalgic for you wasn't it, Dave," Larry said.

Right after Larry's question, another Metro Mobility van pulled up. It looked like one that could hold all three of us. An energetic black man came from behind the wheel. He made the uniform look good, and he had a big smile on his face as he declared, "Gentlemen, are you looking to get back to Courage Center"

We gave an affirmative answer. This guy was courteous and treated us more like human beings than the Metro Mobility driver who brought us to the movies. The loading went smooth as silk. The driver was fast but courteous as we went from the open air to the tight space of the van. I said a prayer that I would get home soon to get my medication. I was tired, and I learned at least a little bit about being in a wheelchair.

Chapter 24

Steve and Julie

"Some friends bring rain on us, but a true friend is more loyal than a brother" (Proverbs 18:24).

I met Julie years ago doing retreats for youth. I always liked her zeal for the Catholic faith that was paired with happy and gentle spirit. She is married to Steve who is a quadriplegic. He has family ties to the Montgomery–Le Center area. He is in a wheelchair due in part to a mistake he made. That was a long time ago, and he is not a bitter man. Instead he is talkative and possesses a servant's heart. He does the best he can with skills he has. The first time they came to visit me was in the later part of my stay at Regency. Julie led the way, being short in stature with brown hair and glasses and a smile that was priceless. We greeted each other. Steve was in a black wheelchair. He had short curly blonde hair and dark-framed glasses. He looked genuinely happy to see me and said, "Hey Dave, Mary Jo told us you would be here." He referred to his aunt who helped raise him and who is a parishioner at Most Holy Redeemer. Mary Jo had always been good to me with her inviting smile or her generous food offerings of hearty soup or sweet cookies. Mary Jo is a giving person, and I can only imagine the role she played in Steve's life. Steve with a look of concern in his eyes said, "Do they have any idea why this happened to you?"

"No, they tell me things that didn't cause it like getting a flu shot or have a long lingering viral illness. They appear to be stumped."

"Wow, that's something. Are you completely paralyzed?"

"I've almost no movement in my legs, but I am starting to be able to move my arms." I lifted my arms a little to show them. "I can't grip much yet, so I'm still being fed, but I'm on full food."

"At least you've the joy of eating."

What I've always like about Julie and Steve is that they are the same age as I am. I think we all graduated high school the same year. Julie and Steve got together long after Steve was in his accident, and they didn't get married until their late thirties. We grew up with the same music and see the world in much the same way.

"You seem to be making progress." Julie said. I knew in my heart this was far better than the drug-induced coma in the intensive care room I had faced not too many days before.

"I am, and it's amazing. I wake up each morning being able to do a little more each day. I don't like being here, but I want to get better."

"After my accident, I spent some time right next store at Courage Center." Steve said with some excitement in his voice.

"Courage Center is my goal. I hope to move there soon."

Julie held up brightly colored solid flags that are made of cloth, shaped like a rectangle and held together on a white cord. Julie explained she made them with their adopted daughter, Jayda, at a camp they went to this summer. She was a young teen originally from India. I hadn't met her, but her proud mom had told me volumes. Julie and Steve are life-giving people. The flags were said to bring good fortune according to the culture in India that was the theme of the camp for families who have an adopted child from India. I thanked her for the flags that helped cheer up my room. We continued to talk for a while until they bid me farewell.

About a week after I moved to Courage Center, they visited. I liked the fact they came in the evening because I was freer to visit. They both worked, she as a pediatric respiratory therapist and he as an insurance agent, so an evening was also good for them. The only drawback to an evening visit was that I was pretty tired. Seeing them warmed my heart, and I had a sudden shot of adrenalin.

"How are you liking your new digs?" Julie said.

"I like it here. The staff's so good. It makes a difference, I think, because I am still making a bunch of progress."

"This place has really changed since I was here," Steve said.

I am pleased this alum is glad to be back at his old recovery environment. Even though I was tired, I offered to show them around. I was excited to show off my surroundings with someone who once knew this place well. Just before we went, Julie pointed out that Jayda's Indian flags made it to my new location. She helped transfer me to my chair and commented about how strong I am getting

"That chair is pretty old school," Steve said.

"Yes it is. My therapist told me they gave me an old one because I wouldn't' be in it very long."

"That's cool."

We made our way through Tou's side of the room and found ourselves out in the hall, and we headed down to the left. We bypassed the elevators and moved to the hallway that leads to the public part of the center. We looked down to the lower level and saw my therapy gym and cafeteria. We passed by the gym where guys were making the floor squeak as they played wheelchair basketball. We stopped for a few minutes outside the door.

"I tried that when I was here and was no good at it. Of course I was never good at basketball before the accident, either," Steve said. This caused all three of us to laugh. "Boy, this place brings back memories. I remember we used to be able to take the elevator up to the roof and smoke." Julie shoots Steve a look of embarrassment, but it soon changes to a smile.

"Well, I don't plan to go to the roof or light up any-time soon," I said with a tease in my voice and again we laughed.

"You look beat, Dave." Julie said. The adrenaline was wearing off, and I started to flatten out as some anima-tion left me. I needed to rest. Julie asked me about get-ting me out of Courage Center, so I could visit them. The thought of going to their house had made me beam. I knew it will be very accessible on account of Steve. We ended our time together with some laughter and promised to stay in touch.

A little over a week later, Julie came by to pick me up for my outing to their house. We were glad to see each other as I transferred easily into her PT Cruiser. The traffic wasn't bad as we make our way across town. Julie said, "Steve is super happy you are able to make it."

"I'm so grateful that you are picking me up."

"No problem. Steve is making ribs. He really likes doing it. He loves to cook and even more to entertain. I some-times have to help out, but he can do most of it."

"That's cool. I can't wait to taste them. Nothing like a good slab of meat."

"Now you sound like Steve," she said with a laugh.

We made our way to their brown Rambler. There was a van in the garage and another small car parked in the driveway away from the garage doors. Looking in the garage doors, I saw a ramp I could enter with my wheelchair.

"I see Betty's already here," Julie said. Betty is her mother. I enjoyed Betty, and I knew her from the retreats as well. She is one cool widow. Once in the house, Betty and I visited a bit.

I looked into the dining room and saw a set of glass doors that led to the deck near the far side of the table. Steve worked over a hot grill from his wheelchair. He saw me and motioned for me to come out there. Julie opened the door to the deck for me.

I rolled out to see Steve on the deck. He working over a silver two-burner grill. I commented on how much I like his BBQ apparatus. Steve smiled and said, "She's my pride and joy . . . next to Julie, of course." We shared a laugh. Steve was amazing as he scooped up the ribs tongs and placed them into a nearby pan. He looked like he might have needed help, but he was steady and overcame obstacles. I was sure he overcame so many difficulties before.

We moved inside, and before we knew it, we were sitting down to a hearty and great-tasting meal. This is almost overwhelming—sharing food and friendship. Even in a warm and wonderful moment such as this, small voices can creep in telling me I don't deserve this. Sometimes when I look at myself, I can only see my imperfections. I needed to be in the imperfect present. This was where God comes into a situation. Steve and Julie were messengers of God's love. I think about how fortunate I am to have friends that will take me in. This reconnection may have not taken place if it were not for GBS. Friendship was reignited due to a horribly debilitating illness. I'm so grateful to enjoy them as friends.

Chapter 25

Carol and the WCC Visit

"To equip the holy ones for work of ministry. To build up the body of Christ" (Ephesians 4:12).

I t was 7:15 a.m., and I was ready. Most days I slept until nine, but this Sunday morning I was cleaned up and waiting. The aide even gave me a little breakfast, and the nurse packed up my pills. I was going to be on a day away. Carol Weiers was going to pick me up and bring me to Masses at the Western Catholic Community, which consisted of my two churches St. John the Evangelist and St. Scholastica. We would make about half the 8 a.m. mass at St. Scholastica and then go to St. John for the 10 a.m. It was October, and I had not been at these churches since early August—two and a half months since I had seen most of my people. Some had visited, but I didn't have contact with most. Certainly I was in their prayers, but now we would be reunited if even for a brief moment.

Carol, a tall woman with light brown hair and glasses, came to my door. She is a very welcoming and hard-working person with a big heart. She was here to drive me and be my aide during this outing. Even though I had started using my walker, we thought it be best to take the wheelchair as it would be easier on me during the long periods of greeting people. Both churches were wheelchair accessible, so I would be able to roll right in. I would find out what it was like to attend mass wheelchair bound.

Carol rolled me out into the fresh morning air. The weather was nice, but fall mornings could be a little brisk. Besides a morning greeting, we had said little when we were exiting Courage Center. Even though I arose early by my standards, I was fully awake and eager with anticipation. Carol seemed a little tired, but she was still her chipper self. "Are you ready for this?" she said.

"I think so. I hardly slept. I'm pretty nervous."

"No need to be nervous. I know they will be glad to see you. I didn't tell very many people you were coming, so it will be a surprise."

"Surprises are fun. I can't wait to see them."

"You have been gone a long time, and people miss you. Fr. Roger is good, but he is not you."

Carol helped me transfer into the passenger's front seat of her white SUV. With relative ease, she folded up my chair and placed it in the back of her vehicle. In few moments, we were on the open road. The cities whizzed by, and soon we were among the more open areas near Shakopee as we traveled down 169. I wanted to see the open fields. I had been to Joan's church a few times and out a few other times, but I longed for the open spaces.

The fields with crops were nearing harvest time. It was such a privilege to view the bounty of the land. I tried to think about how doing therapy was bringing a bounty to my recovery. I was elated to view the beauty of fall.

We arrived at St. Scholastica after mass had begun. Carol pushed me up the ramp, and we were in the building just after consecration where the bread and wine became the Body and Blood of Christ. Through the people, I saw Fr. Roger in green vestments standing behind the altar that was enclosed in a wood railing that served as a support for the former pastor, Fr. Richard Rodel, who passed away the previous summer. Deacon Bob Wagner was standing behind and off to the left in his bright green stole over his right shoulder. The church seated about 200, and there were around 110 or so, who knelt with their backs to me. It is a nice crowd in their wooden pews. Two altar servers in white robes with brown ropes about their waists knelt in front of the altar on the edge of a blue-and-red patterned carpet with white fringe, lying a step down from the altar level. Off to the left, there were two chairs, one red and the other green. On either side of them were two red-cushioned stools that matched the red chair. The legs of the stools and the legs and arms of the chairs were a beautiful tan wood. Off to the right was a brown wooden pulpit raised up a step, so it can be seen from a distance. The walls of the sanctuary was painted light blue with white mixed in making it resemble sky. There was a Holy Spirit window up high in the middle. It looked a little grimy, but it actually was painted with some light brown tones.

A few people in back saw me and extended silent greetings. More people saw me as they came back from communion. There was a hushed excitement as I sat in my wheelchair. Near the end of mass, just before the final blessing, Fr. Roger said with his booming voice, "Fr. Dave is here. Be sure to greet him in the back."

Many heads turned with big smiles. After the ministers left the sanctuary, there was a steady stream of people coming up me in the wheelchair. As I look back, I can't link comments with individual people, nor could I attempt to say what response I gave them. It is a blur—a nice soothing blur, but a blur nonetheless. So I remember things like, "So glad you made it here, Father."

"You look so good."

"We hope you make it back soon."

"Father, I bet we could prop you up there, and you could say mass right now."

I took the compliments in. I couldn't think of much of a reply, so I said things like, "Thank you."

"Glad to be here."

"Glad to be seen."

I was so thrilled to be with all these people. This experience made me want to try even harder to get better. I get a good view of the Immaculate Heart of Mary Statue as Carol rolled me out the south door on to the ramp. I was tired, but I realized I have one more church to go.

The drive between Heidelberg and Union Hill is about six miles, and I could do this drive in my sleep. Wonderful rural scenes mark both sides of the road with a few farmsteads and a few more houses out in the country. The green of summer turned to the pale browns of fall. Captivated by the view, I looked out the window of Carol's SUV. I took this beauty all in as I really missed seeing all of this country. Carol breaks the silence, "How are you doing?"

"Great, just a little lost in thought."

"I bet this is a little overwhelming."

"You are right about that."

"Did you notice Barton's pumpkins opening up again?"

"Yes, the patch is so great every year."

"They are donating a few pumpkins and gourds to decorate church."

Fran Barton, the matriarch of the pumpkin patch, is a very strong parishioner. Along with her wonderful family, she has a multigenerational pumpkin patch for the community. I hoped to see her at the upcoming mass.

We drove right into Union Hill that sprawls out a little bit on both sides of the highway. On the north, there is a beautiful ballpark. There are also a few houses along with the Union Hill Bar. The church is right across the highway, along with a few more houses. Isn't that what every small town needs—a church and a bar? I have heard many a story about people, including priests, being among the first to make the journey to the bar after mass. I have had a few burgers there and even one small funeral luncheon.

The church is actually on Hub drive, a frontage road off 19 that is nonexistent for most GPS systems. I was dropped at the north-facing door that let me roll right into the church with no steps. There is a little space on the north side near the door that goes to the front of the seating for the congregation. Across the church is a door that leads to a sidewalk that connects the old school building, still used for meetings and weekly faith formation classes. The other door is in the rear of the church to the west. There are two steps that lead you out to the county road that separates the church from the cemetery.

From my view in front of church, I am comforted by the statue of St. John the Evangelist on the high altar that is a beautiful white structure that also hold St. Francis to the north and St. Anthony to the south. The walls are decorated with scenes from the life of Jesus and his closest followers. The altar to the Blessed Virgin Mary was right in front of me, and I looked off to my right and saw Fr. Roger, Deacon Bob, and four servers enter the sanctuary. The mass was an excellent prayer for me here as I am up front and lost in the ecstasy of the ritual. The Word of God was spoken, and Fr. Roger gave a nice homily. Then came the Liturgy of the Eucharist in which we received the Body and Blood of Jesus. I remember the host coming right to me, and I was really caught up in receiving Jesus. In communion, I realized people saw me at the mass, and I received a lot of taps on the shoulder and mouthed well wishes from people on their way back from communion.

At the end of mass, Carol wheeled me outside to the back door of the church, so I was there to see the people come out. It was a glorious series of well wishes, not unlike at St. Scholastica. I felt so cared for and longed to be back in ministry. After greeting people, I rolled into the office and saw Donnie, one of my favorite guys. He is a tall senior citizen who wears a ball cap everywhere but in church. "There's Father; he's the best."

"Thanks, Donnie, but I'm not the one who has a baseball field named after me." We laughed, but it is true that last summer they named the field at Union Hill Park, Don Giesen Field. He started there during his baseball career and took care of that field almost his whole life. Donnie has visited me a few times, so we had kept up with each other. He had been sick a number of times, so he knew what I was going through. Being tired didn't overshadow my motivation to get better.

Chapter 26

Don and the Mass

"After he had given thanks, he broke the bread and said, 'Take this all of you. This is my body that is for you. Do this in memory of me'" (1 Corinthians 11:24).

He was on his way. Fr. Don DeGrood, my priesthood classmate and good friend was coming to see me. I was really missing him as I hadn't seen him since well before the illness. In fact, I can't even remember when we had been in touch before I went in. He called to apologize he hadn't come to see me, but now he was coming at a great time to see visitors. Just a few minutes later, I heard a firm knock on the door to my room. "Hey Don, is that you? Come right in."

I hear the whoosh of the dividing curtain and I see a familiar face. Don is about five feet, ten inches, and thin. He has curly brown hair and a big smile on his face. Don has good energy about him, and he has always been a positive person in my life. "Brother, it is so good to see you. I bring greetings from guys who are praying for you." Don was smiling and holding a bag under his arm.

"It looks like you brought the stuff for Mass." I hadn't said mass all this time, and was looking forward to offering mass since Don brought it up on the phone. I kept praying during my illness, but I missed the mass. Celebrating the mass is so vital to being a priest. As the Second Vatican Council from the 1960s put it, "Eucharist is the source and summit of the faith."

We used the conference room just next store. I wheeled ahead into this room with a big conference table and quite a few chairs. It had a bit of an industrial look, but it would become a cathedral for us as we offered the Holy Mass.

"I had my care conference here last week."

"How did it go?"

"Real well, they said I was a rock star."

"I guess that is good," he said with a smile.

We used the table as the altar. Don got out a small cup called a chalice that he screwed the base into the cup part. He had a paten or small plate that he used for two small pieces of unleavened bread called hosts. There was a small container of wine and one of water. Don subscribed to a magazine that contained the scripture readings for the first part of mass and the words of the Roman Missal for the opening prayer and the second part of the mass where bread and wine become the Body and Blood of Jesus.

"Would you like to celebrate or concelebrate? Whatever you feel more comfortable doing."

"I'll concelebrate." I was a bit nervous having never celebrated for over two months. Don would celebrate, meaning he would take the lead on the prayers of the priest. I would take a less active role as concelebrant, but it would be my way of offering the mass as well.

Don took a white robe called an alb. He placed it around my upper body and let the lower part of the alb go around my chair. He put a long, thin, white sturdy piece of cloth around my neck called a stole. The colors usually correspond with the color of the season, but white can always be used. The color white often signifies special occasions, and in my mind this was indeed a very special occasion. He dressed similarly, and we began reciting our common prayers and reading the scriptures of the day. The Catholic Church has readings for every day of the year. Don let me read the passage from St. Paul's letter to the Romans. I let the words flow off my tongue as the reading was an intimate form of prayer. Next I read one of the 150 psalms, complete with an antiphon between the psalm's verses. Don read the Gospel passages. This is taken from the writings of the one of the Evangelists: Matthew, Mark, Luke, or John. He then gave a small reflection called a homily. I didn't remember a word he said, but having him preach was just so heartwarming.

I could smell a hint of industrial cleaner and a bit of air freshener. Churches sometimes smell of wood and perhaps the faint scent of incense. We didn't have that smell, but I tried to imagine that we were in one of my small churches with that pleasant scent. The shades were drawn on the windows, but the lighting was so

good that I imagined being in bright sunshine. The light
of the experience was glowing even if the outside might
have been darkening. The slight hum of the lights was
blending with Don's soothing voice.

We then got ready to turn the bread and wine into the
Body and Blood of Jesus. When we reached the most
sacred part of the mass, Don and I said together, "Take
this, all of you, and eat of it; this is my body given up
for you." Don raised the host up and paused for prayer.
Don then genuflected and I lowered my head in rever-
ence for the host we believe went from mere bread to
the Body of Christ.

Then Don held the chalice, or crafted metal cup, and
we said these words, "Take this all of you and drink of
it for this is the chalice of my blood, the blood of the
new and eternal covenant, offered for you and for many
for the forgiveness of sins. Do this in memory of me."

Don raised up the chalice and paused for prayer. I was
in thankful prayer for the miracle that was happening
before us. Then he placed it on the table and genuflected on his right knee. I bowed my head as I remained
in my chair.

Don went on to pray to the Father about Jesus and
the Holy Spirit. He prayed for Pope Benedict and our
Archbishop John Neinstedt. He prayed for the dead
along with our Blessed Mother Mary and all the saints
who have gone before us in faith. The prayers were finished up with us praying together, "Through him with

him and in him, in O God almighty Father in the unity of the Holy Spirit, one God forever and ever. Amen."

We then prayed the Our Father and shared a sign of peace by. Don broke one of the hosts in half and placed a small piece of the host into the chalice of wine turned precious blood, uniting Body and Blood. We both consumed the Body and Blood of Christ in the form of bread and wine. It looks like bread and wine, smells like bread and wine, and tastes like bread and wine, but by our faith, we believe it is the Body and Blood of Jesus. This was all that really mattered.

I was so happy to receive Jesus, and to receive it with Don made it even better. I had been away from this experience, and now I was able to say mass as a priest again. This was another step in an exciting progression of making it back to normal. I felt energized by the mass and told Don he would have to come back soon. I was so happy he came to visit. I did not receive many priest visitors, but some used my CaringBridge or sent letters, such as "One of those emails went out, asking for prayers for you. Guys are asking about you. They are concerned."

Some have called and sent cards. Joe and Creags came when I was at my last hospital. It was so good to see them. Fr. Joseph Gallatin and Fr. Michael Creagan are also classmates of ours. They visited me at Regency, bringing some inspirational pictures of Jesus and Mary. I brought those pictures with me to Courage Center. It is nice to have religious items in a secular world. It made me proud to be a Catholic priest. Now I had celebrated

Mass and would be able to do so again soon. Different chaplains, both priest and lay, have made sure I got communion most weeks, but it was really special to celebrate my own mass. I could really feel the brotherhood of the priesthood.

The adrenalin of this incredible event and all the other things I had done that day was starting to wear off. I was extremely tired. Don pushed me the short distance to my room. We said good night, and he promised to come again.

About a week later, he did come. This time I was the celebrant, and it was again a life-giving mass. I reflected on how important mass is and how I longed to be celebrating it on a regular basis soon. The mass is a service to the people, but it is also spiritually and emotionally who I was as a priest.

Chapter 27

Six-Minute Walk

"Your Word is a lamp for my feet and a light for my path" (Psalm 119:105).

I n a session with Tina, I was having trouble using a cane. I just couldn't get a rhythm with it. Tina looked at me from a few feet away and said, "You don't need that silly cane."

"Are you sure? I don't want to fall."

"I don't want you to fall, either, but you have better balance than you think"

"If you say so, I will try and trust."

"Yes, you must try and trust yourself."

She brought me over to the raised mat, and I sat down. She took the cane away and had me stand back up. I did a little wobble as I quickly caught my balance as Tina gave me a little reassurance as she held on to my safety belt. After stabilizing, I started taking steps again. From that point on, I never used a cane or walker in therapy again. I would use the walker outside of therapy, but that was only a precaution if I didn't have a therapist ready to catch me with a safety belt.

I really liked therapy. I loved how Tina pushed me, and I felt that I had some chemistry with her. This allowed me to maximize my sessions and worked toward a greater connection with my mind, body, and spirit. Tina had a look on her face that showed she wanted to challenge me; the

"While you're fresh, I'm going to have you do something called the six-minute walk test. You are going to walk any way you can. The faster the better as you will be accessed by the distance you cover." Tina gave me just a little bit of assistance as we made it out to the hallway just outside the Creekside gym. Once I was stabilized, she looked at her stop watch and said, "Go"

This started me ambling down the hallway. I tried to go as rapidly as I could. We headed down the hallway and went into the dining room. I made it through there and went down the hall past the Gardenview gym that I had used a few times. We continued down the hallway into where the ground floor residents lived. I knew some of them, but often the floors kept to themselves. Actually, it was truer that I kept to myself. I would reach out to a few people, but often it wasn't returned much. I am not sure if it was because I was a priest, older, rapidly getting better, or some other reason. I just knew that most folks didn't talk to me much. I had a few lunch table friends and my roommate, but it was hard to get better when most were not. This made me not want to tell of my progress. I had a lot of support, including staff.

"Keep going; you are doing great." Tina's words motivated me to keep putting one foot in front of the other.

"Dave, you are walking!" These were the words of Tou, my roommate. I was so tired that I didn't have the breath to answer back. I smiled at him, and he smiled back. I went past him at a rate I thought was fast, but I am sure that it wasn't so fast.

"Push it. You are getting toward the end. Just a little more," Tina said, and these words encouraged me. I tried to reach deep inside to use all of my energy to travel farther. "OK, you can stop now."

Out of breath, I wobbled a bit, and Tina grabbed my belt and steadied me into a nearby chair. I was so tired, and my lungs and my legs start to burn. It felt good to be done. "OK, you stay here, and I will go back and measure the distance."

I nodded as I continued to breathe heavy. I saw my Aunt Susan with her sister and her sister's husband, Craig, who was also a resident.

"I saw you walking," my aunt said joyfully.

"Six minutes' worth," I said back, still a little out of breath.

"That sounds pretty tough, but you made it."

"He certainly did." Tina said from around the corner as she appears holding a measuring wheel that paced out my steps. She pulled a calculator from her pocket. "Give me a sec, and I will figure out a percentage of how fast you were going according with someone of your age group should go." She punches a few numbers and comes up with a total. "You are 48 and with the distance you covered you are about at 48 percent."

"How is that? Is it fast enough?"

"Not bad, but you might struggle making it across the street at a light."

"We only have two stoplights in the town I work in, and I don't go through them much on foot."

"Well, we will have you try it again as I know you will do better as your stamina increases."

I am getting pretty comfortable in this chair, and my breathing is back to normal.

"Let's hit the stairs as I want you to lift a few weights:

"Can't we take the elevator?" I said in jest.

"You really didn't ask that, did you?" she slyly said back with a tease in her voice.

We approached the stairs, and I got ready to climb. They were tough, but with the railing I did pretty well. This was great practice because I will have steps in my parent's house. I made it up the multistep climb broken up by a landing. I was again a little out of breath. We left the industrial-like staircase for the bright, warm first floor. If we went to the right, we would go past the elevator into my residence floor. Instead, we went left into a brick hallway area, passing by the clinic entrance on the left, down the hallway to the weight room.

"OK, let's see what those legs are made of." Tina said this with authority as she led me into the corner to the dreaded leg press machine. I was thinking that it might be a little much, but I have learned to put my brain on and moved forward with a positive frame of mind. I saw other patient/physical therapist duos around the room. There was also a few brawny guys trying to get a good workout in. I felt more confident around so many people who tried to get the maximum strength out of their bodies. I gingerly approached the machine as I went and sat in the machine and lay on my back. I placed my feet with my knees bent on the large metal plate before me. I looked and saw my feet pointing out in a "V." This was common for me. This "V" position seemed to be the new normal. My therapist and I were both displeased by this. The "V" is normal for one who craved safety because the position was more stable. I was on safety mode 24/7. I wish I could have been a little less safe, but until then, all I can do was try to correct it. Tina knew this process as it presented itself time and time again. So she just gently said, "Feet." I went ahead and made the adjustment and moving my feet felt forced, but I knew this was for my own good. Once I made the adjustment, she said, "There you go; that is more like it. Now let's see what you can do." I couldn't see where she put the weight pin, but I knew

Tina would set me up for failure. The weight went up easy. "Give me ten of those"

"This isn't bad," I said as I pushed with a steady motion.

"I will give you more weight. Just keep pushing, though. I hope you are counting because I'm not. I do think you are getting close."

"That makes ten."

She pulled out the pin and placed it in again. I can hear the metal strike the metal. She looked me in the eyes with a smile and said, "There you go. This won't be as easy, but I know you can do it."

I pushed again, and I called upon my legs to make the same motion. She was right as this weight was much harder. My push was shaky, but the weight went up. I counted out loud this time, so there wouldn't be any doubt.

As I finished, Tina smiled and said, "Alright, good one. You got one more in you?"

I nodded and saw her adjust the pin one more time. I pushed harder this time. My two legs were like pistons pushing in a well-oiled machine. Even though this weight was heavier I regained my form. The strain caused me to be silent this time, but Tina started to count out loud,

"That makes ten. How do you feel?"

"My legs are rubbery, but I'm happy."

"You should be. Now let's do two more machines and call it a day."

We worked on my upper body. These are hard, but my upper body has regained much of its strength, so these machines were easier. I liked to work out my legs, but this change was a welcome break.

"OK, Dave, you worked hard. Would you like the elevator, or can you take on the stairs?"

"Bring on the stairs."

"That was a bit of a trick question, and as per usual you have chosen wisely."

I welled up with a little pride, and I moved down the hall with authority. I knew the stairs were a challenge I could handle. Going down the steps was actually harder. It wouldn't seem that way because you were going downhill, but going down took more muscle control. I thanked God for the railing as I plodded down one step and then another. I made the landing with ease. This last set was difficult, but I pressed on. I went through the door that led to the hallway. My session was over, and I gathered up my walker and headed back to my room. This time I took the elevator.

Chapter 28

The Nurse from Indiana

"To be a minister of Christ Jesus to the gentiles in performing the priestly service of the Gospel of God" (Romans 15:16).

There was a Courage Center nurse that I was fond of. Amanda wasn't very experienced; in fact, I believe this was her first job, and she started a month or two before I got there. She was a RN and still in her early to mid-twenties. She was about five feet, seven inches, and slender. She had chestnut brown hair she usually wore in a ponytail, and she also had crystal blue eyes. She had a very small, pointy nose, and her completion had a few freckles. I would have been proud to call her a daughter. This wasn't because of her outer beauty but because of the beautiful heart she possessed. She was so conscientious, always getting things done quickly. If she made a promise to return, she was timely about it. She made you feel like you were the most important person she was dealing with that day. Amanda did things with great joy and with an understanding way beyond her years. She was a good conversationalist, talking of medicine, sports, and current events.

My priesthood has been rewarding, but from time to time I have experiences that make me long for biological fatherhood. Amanda brought up those kind of feeling with in me. She was around the same age as the brides I worked with in preparing them for marriage.

One evening when Amanda popped in, I decided to try and pay her a compliment. "How's the best nurse at Courage Center?"

"You have to ask her when you see her." This was her humble reply that made me think even higher of her.

Amanda is just one example of the caring people I interacted with during my hospital stays. I have always been a little fascinated with the medical field, and I have a great deal of respect for the men and women who work in the industry. My job has some similarities, especially when I worked with the sick and the dying. This gave me energy and a deep appreciation for the sanctity of life. Whoever ministers, whether one was a health care worker or as a religious leader, we deal with family systems.

She came to check on me. She had a good habit of just poking her head in a number of times each shift. She was always doing something for me.

"My boyfriend got a job here."

"So you found one here, too."

"Yes, he knows a few people around here, and I am meeting so many people."

"Where about do you live?"

"We got a place just north of the cities near Ramsey."

"So you live with your boyfriend?" I said gingerly.

"I do, and I suppose you think that is bad," she said with a little sadness in her voice.

"It is not my first hope," I said. I hoped she wouldn't feel judged when I said that. I was only concerned for her.

"I'm not that happy about it, either. I believe we should be married if we live together, but I don't really know anybody around here to live with."

Amanda's usually perky demeanor changed, with her eyes looking downcast, and she had the presence of worry lines on her forehead.

"It sounds like it is hard for you. I don't bring it up to condemn you but to look out for you."

She nods and looks at me with those big eyes that look as if they want to tear up. "I love him and I think he loves me, and I do wish we could marry."

"You should let him know how you feel."

"I try, but he always changes the subject."

"Why do you think he does that?"

As I posed this question, the smile came back to her face. She got a little gleam in her eyes, and she answered in an excited voice like this was going to be a new revelation. "I think he is scared!"

Communication is so important for all relationships. Amanda seemed to have made a breakthrough. Her boyfriend is going through something that is all too common for people in his generation. From what Amanda told me, he was afraid of commitment. Young people these days are finding it harder to commit. They are marrying older and waiting to have children.

We had a moment of silence as I watched Amanda process. She is a bright young woman who was convicted with a keen sense of right and wrong. I was certain she came from a loving family, and she probably had good modeling from her parents. I think Amanda wanted to do the right thing, but she is most likely afraid she will push him away. This is a real problem, and I couldn't solve it in a few minutes. I just wanted her to think about her life and hope she was able to rely on what seemed to be a well-developed conscience.

"Can I pray for you?"

"Absolutely. I can tell you are a man of faith." She perked back up with her warm and friendly smile. Her face was narrow but really expressive. Her mood was often on display. She was fun to be around, and I was sure she could make friends easily. She very sweetly asked if I needed anything else. When I said no, she was gone in a flash.

The Catholic Church teaches that a couple should not live together before marriage. This might seem outdated, but the Church sides with the woman. It wants to make sure the woman is protected should she lose her living arrangement as many times the lease or ownership might be in his name. Should a breakup occur, she could be out with very little to show for it. Even if where they live is in both of their names, things may get bitter if there is a parting of ways. If someone is married, there is at least the process of divorce that tries to work these things out.

I know people want to try out marriage and think that living together is a way to make sure. Studies show that really isn't the case because marriage is much more permanent. There is much more of a connection when someone becomes legally and sometimes religiously connected in the bond of matrimony. This is a delicate issue. All pastoral matters should be dealt with individually, with as much care as possible.

I reflected on our brief conversation and wondered if I should have brought it up. She seemed to be a young woman of high morals, and with minimum prompting, she basically was hard on herself. She went from caregiver to a sort of care receiver if even for a moment. She knew where I stood, and I believe she respected me for that. During these three months, I received a whole lot of care. For I could do nothing on my own. It felt real good to give a little back. I longed to be a caregiver again.

I also love that God made me a spiritual father of many. I have been able to have an impact on people I have barely known. Priesthood has been a rewarding life for me. Being able to befriend people of different generations is something I love to try and do. Amanda was my nurse, but she also let me see her as a person as well. I will forever cherish this. This conversation brought us closer together. This connection was near the end of my stay, and I never asked if she talked to her boyfriend or not. I didn't really think it was my place. I was just in the business of planting seeds and nurturing those who ask for help. Amanda and I had a few more nights together, and the last night ended with a big hug.

Amanda was a big help in my healing process. I think I had a few doubts about whether I would be able to return to ministry. When one is sick, there is so much self-focus. My time with Amanda showed me I could reach out more. We had many conversations before this one that built up enough trust for us to broach a tender topic like this. She trusted me, and I believe she knew I was concerned for her. Having conversations like this is risky, but I believe reaching out is so important. God made us for human interaction.

Chapter 29

Why walk When You Can Run?

"Do you not know that the runners in the stadium all run in the race, but only one wins the prize? Run so as to win." (1 Corinthians 9:24).

On my second to the last day at Courage Center I had my last physical therapy session with Tina. She was dressed in black, and she had a smile that lit up the room.

"Last session, are you excited?"

"I will miss this place, but I am ready to move on."

"Let's start with stairs, move to weights, and then I have a special surprise for you."

"Wow, I look forward to it all!"

"That is a great attitude, and I am going to miss it. I will give you a card with my email. I want updates. I want to hear all you do in therapy. You are all set up in Northfield, aren't you?"

I thought about the future. I would be going to outpatient therapy, and I was excited. Being outpatient, this therapy might not be as intense, but I will be expected to do some on my own. That is why this getting a home program is so important. I would only work with a volunteer twice while trying to master the program. I was excited to have a strong home program. I wanted to finish my time at Courage Center with a bang.

"Let's go tackle those stairs."

We walked out of Creekside gym and went to the familiar staircase. I had worked these stairs a number of times. I even made it once to the third floor, which made four flights. It was a workout, but it felt good. Climbing steps is such a basic thing most people take for granted. I was now relearning that skill. As I gripped the rail to go, I realized that I didn't have the death grip that I once had. This grip was much more natural. After a while, I would be able to go up without a rail. In fact, if there is one available I will probably always lightly use it. It would be quite some time before stair climbing would be as automatic as it once was. This task required much effort, but I was holding my own. I climbed these steps with vigor on my fresh legs.

We went into the weight room, and as we had most of the time, we started with a warm up. I first tackled the elliptical machine. Tina braced me as I tried to climb on mostly under my own power.

"There you go, Dave. Let's try seven minutes."

"You got it," I said as my legs started to pump. I even used the arms this time. I was amazed at how easy it was. Seven minutes were completed in no time. I knew I could do more, but there was so much I wanted to do. Next, we shifted to the treadmill.

"OK, Dave, this will be easy for you, too. I want you to concentrate on striking with your heels. You sometimes tend to let the front of your foot come down first. I know you can do this. Concentrate now, and in no time it will come naturally."

"If you say so."

"I do and you can too. Attitude is everything."

The treadmill actually came pretty easy on that last day. Things were going like a dream. We flew off the treadmill after it stopped right into a number of weights that tested my upper body and then worked to strengthen different parts of my legs. I looked around the weight room, realizing this was perhaps my last time in here. I reflected on all the progress I have made. I was really pumped to do weights.

We ventured down the hall to the gym in the public part of Courage Center. I had been there before with Tou to watch wheelchair rugby. Tou was considering joining, and I was with to see him check out in a return trip to this high-energy area. The spirited competitors practiced 3-on-3 drills, trying to move a ball into a goal. There was quite a bit of slamming going on as they battled in modified chairs with big metal wheels. The sound made the impacts sound severe, but the reality is that it was not very punishing as they wore padding, and most of them had limited feeling in their legs. This gladiator-like action still seemed to take much skill, and I was not about to try it. This wasn't a sport for the faint of heart. These guys were athletes with large amounts of upper body strength to compensate for the lack of use of their legs. Tou appeared to be warming up to the possibility, but I am not sure if he ever took the guys up on this seemingly tough activity. The sport also looked pretty fun.

Now the gym was quiet as Tina and I entered alone. This was a hardwood floor with a basketball goal on each end. The cement walls were white with plenty of blue padding along the two ends under the baskets. There were black and red stripes on the shiny floor, and our shoes made quiet, squeaking noises as we walked to the center of the gym. With minimal instruction, Tina put me through a number of balance drills just like the ones we had done in the hallways outside of Creekside. They were a little trickier here as the walls were much further apart and even though there was an assurance having Tina near. There was a greater danger in falling. That was one of the fears that was fortunately never fully realized. I was crossing over my feet, trying to walk toe to toe along with walking forward, backward, and sideways. These were all pretty good tricks. Their success met with smiles and encouragement from Tina. Then she gave a dramatic pause and standing before me she said, "OK, Dave, we are going to try something. I am going to stand behind you with this band, and you are going to run."

I look at her a bit dazed. I could barely walk as it was and had to use a walker in public. This crazy therapist was now going to have me do something that I hadn't done proficiently in years. I could tell she thought I could do it, so I supposed I could suspend imagination and give it a shot.

"How are you doing? Do you want to try this?"

"I think so," I said with a shaky voice.

"I never ask you to do something I didn't think you could handle. I promise you won't fall. I will be right there." This sounded reassuring. Tina came around behind me with the tubing around my waist. She gave me just the right amount of space. This felt a bit awkward, but I braced for my best shot. "1, 2, 3, Go!" My legs started to churn, but I struggled to get a little speed. I was reassured by the strap around my waist, and I really felt balanced. "You don't have to go fast, but I want you see what it is like to let both feet leave the ground."

I placed the thought in my head, and I visualized myself doing it. Things slowed down, and suddenly I was running. I have run 5Ks before, but now I feel like I am training for the marathon of life. I hadn't experienced this feeling in years, but now I was doing it. I was only going the length of the gym, but it felt like a couple of miles. I got lost in the moment, and finally Tina brought me back down with "That was really good. Your feet were really leaving the ground."

Tina was praising me, but I barely heard her as I was caught up in the exhilaration of the moment. I was so out of breath I wasn't sure if I could talk at all. I slowed down, and we stopped with Tina braced me. I was both tired and exhilarated. I finally caught my breath and said, "How much will I be able to run?"

"I can see you doing 5Ks again, and I want a video of you finishing your first one. This will depend on your neuropathy. But, hey, for you, the sky is the limit."

Chapter 30

Walking Out

"Nothing gives me greater joy then to have my children walking in the truth" (3 John 4).

The next day, I had a leisurely morning, making sure I was packed and ready to go. Right about noon, I went to eat my final meal at Courage Center. I had this great-looking chicken wrap sandwich and a cup of crème of broccoli soup. I was at a full table of residents, including a nineteen-year-old woman with cerebral palsy. She was delightful with her bob-cut brown hair and big brown eyes. She was in a sophisticated wheelchair that was pink, and she had a huge smile as she fed herself. She was also Catholic, and we had quite a few chats. She was also leaving today, but she already knew she would be back for some more intense therapy in a month. A parishioner gave me a smooth wooden cross to hold in times of pain. I used the cross many times. The only stipulation was that I had to give it away before I left the hospital. I chose to give it to this young woman, and she happily accepted this symbol of what Jesus did for us.

My friend, Mike, with whom I shared most meals, was there. Mike was kind of in a holding pattern as they sought the right housing for him. He was witty, and I would miss him. There were a couple of other women in wheelchairs at our table with various maladies, with whom I was not that familiar. Our meal included a photo-taking session for promotional pictures for Courage Center. I could tell from the angles they were taking that Mike and I weren't in many of the shots. We did all have to sign a waiver when the photos were completed.

Shortly after lunch, I reported to meet with my volunteer who was to go over my home program. He is a real nice kid from St. Thomas University. He looks like he know his way around the weight room. He appears strong, but not real bulky. He had a copy of my exercise program on a clipboard. He smiled and said, "Are you ready for this?"

"You bet."

"Is it true you're a priest?"

"Yes, I am, down in New Prague."

"I know where that is. I like all the priests at St Thomas, and I even took a few theology classes."

"Did you like them?"

"I only took the minimum, but they were pretty cool. I want to be a physical therapist someday."

"I can't say enough about PTs, as I have had nothing but a great experience with all of them."

We were using one of the raised therapy mats. The other therapy mat had quite a crowd. Anna was there with a resident I didn't know very well. She was giving him therapy, and Tina was watching her, and three observers who appeared to be students were listening intently to her as she commented on what Anna was trying to accomplish. I tried not to let this active commotion disturb my exercises. I knew that I was going to need this home program for at least a few days until I get connected in Northfield. Tina said they would modify my exercises to keep me challenged.

We got to the point in my program where I had to do my sit stands. This literally meant I would sit down and stand up quickly. He had me pretty high on the mat, so they were pretty easy. At this point, I was tired, so I didn't correct him. Tina looked over and said, "Hey, get that mat lower. You know better, Dave." she said with a tease in her voice.

"This low?" the Tommie said to me.

"A little lower," I said back.

"That's more like it," Tina said with approval in her voice.

The enthusiastic student continued to put me through the paces, and we finished at about the same time Tina's group broke up. She went ahead of us with her students in tow. I retrieved the new walker that I was now using that came from a friend of my mom. The original "Walker Texas Ranger" was retired. I do have the fancy pouch on the new walker, making it a good stand in. I move to the space outside the therapist's office. I peered in the room and saw Tina. She looked to her students and said something to them in a hushed tone and made her way toward me. "All ready to go, Dave?"

"My parents are probably up in my room waiting for me."

"You put real effort in here at Courage, and I thank you for really working the program."

"You were a big help. You and the other therapists, but it was a lot of you."

"It was really you, and I was glad to help when I was around. Didn't I meet you and turn around and head out of town?"

"That sounds about right, but you were around quite a bit, and you taught me plenty."

"You also taught me, Dave."

We stopped and had a moment, and then Tina initiated a hug. I see Tina as a sister in Christ. Our paths may not cross again, but I have those therapeutic moments to carry me through. There would be challenges ahead on this journey to health. My time with Tina was but one step on the road to recovery.

My time there was coming to an end. I had some rather dramatic good byes. This place really grew on me in a short six weeks. I was hospitalized for three months, and now it was coming to an end. I had these thoughts as I came back from Creekside. As I continue down the hallway to my room at the end of the hall, I saw Marie, the nurse, dressed in her pink scrubs with an unidentified print with dominated by a light blue color. Her almond-shaped Asian face sported a smile as she said, "You ready to leave now?

"Yes, I am."

"I will get your medication and meet you in your room." I realized the end is near as a small tear develops in the corner of my eye.

I made my way to my room and saw my parents on my side. They looked kind of fidgety. They are both wearing light jackets. Seeing their jackets, I wondered what I should wear. As if she was reading my mind my Mom said, "I brought your blue jacket to wear home." Once a mother always a mother, and thank God for that.

My dad looks extra fidgety as he said, "We better get going if we want to miss rush hour."

I glance at my watch and said, "It is still a little before 2. I think we will be fine." He either agrees or he thinks better than arguing with a sick son. I continued, "Besides we have to wait for my nurse to give me my drugs."

"We took most of the stuff, leaving just one bag a piece," Mom said in a proud tone.

They had carried out a couple a loads already as I had accumulated a great deal of stuff after being here six weeks. Just then Marie entered the room. "Well, David, I will go over your prescriptions. There are some extra vitamins that you paid for, but don't take any more. Basically we are giving you all the open drugs you paid for and prescriptions for the next three months or until you meet with your regular doctor."

She reviewed the many drugs I would take. I felt like a test lab rat with all the different stuff I was on—better living through chemistry. What I did learn from previous doctoring is that they know a whole lot more than I do, so I listened to my doctor.

My eyes were glazing over a bit when Marie finished. She looked at me and said, "You have two appointments. One with the PT place in Northfield on Monday and Dr. Warhol the last week in November."

"Dr. Warhol?"

"She like to follow up with all her patients."

"Thanks, Marie. I have enjoyed you as a nurse."

"Take care, David, I am so glad you are getting better." Marie slipped out of the room, and my parents picked up their bags in unison.

"Better get going," Dad said as they both headed out the door. I got up from my chair and positioned my walker in front of me. I made it just outside the door, and I looked back. The room is quite different on each side of the half-drawn curtain. Even though Tou has a disability, he is still a teenager. It was a mess of clothes, medical supplies featuring half tubes of salve and bandage wrappers, candy wrappers, pop cans, and papers from the places we had been, like the movies and the art museum. In Tou's defense some of the mess may have been the aide's fault, and there were times my half wasn't always as neat as a pin.

I looked around my room as it was so bare without my stuff. The plain mattress with no sheets and the empty walls made the room seem so sterile. This half of the room was now ready for the next guy to come in and start working hard. By the sounds of it, there was someone coming in that night. Soon I would be a faded memory. I had suddenly broken from my trance and realized I better try and catch up to my parents.

I took the elevator down to the ground floor and wheeled toward the door. Just then, I thought about what Tina told me about walking out the front door. I was now approaching the front door, and I knew what I was going to do. I took the walker with the bag outside the door. I walked easily back in the hospital on my own. Then I turned and walked back out. I had done what I predicted when I first starting working with Tina six weeks ago. She was like another "Blue Angel." I was proud of my work at Courage Center. I had more therapy ahead, but these were critical steps in my journey of life.

CPSIA information can be obtained
at www.ICGtesting.com
Printed in the USA
FFHW022329091218
49768235-54248FF

9 781545 616581